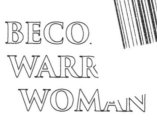

BECO. WARR WOMAN

9 RULES TO SORT YOUR SHIT

JEN WILSON

Published in 2016 by Warrior Woman Media

ISBN Paperback: 978-0-9957070-0-9
Ebook: 978-0-9957070-1-6

A CIP catalogue copy of this book can be
found in the British Library.

Author photograph © Julie Broadfoot

Published with the help of Indie Authors World

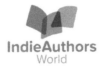

IndieAuthors
World

DEDICATION

To my Soulmates

CHAPTER 1

THE CREATION STORY

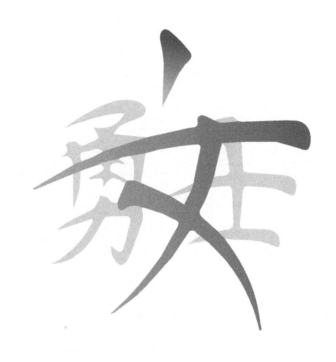

I believe that the ultimate goal in life for us is to be happy and that is why I have written this book "9 Rules to Sort Your Shit" and created an amazing coaching programme for women in the Warrior Woman Project Academy.

There was a time in my life where I felt lost, stuck, and living in Groundhog Day. And when I started working with my coaching clients I discovered that, that is pretty much how they felt too. Or in other words, they felt shit. The fact that you are reading this book suggests you may be in that same place. The good news for you my dear reader is you are not alone.

I have overcome some interesting challenges in my life so far and I am also continually working on the new ones that seem to be thrown my way. These challenges I believe are just to keep us on our toes and keep learning and growing as humans.

The good news for all of us is that we are a lifelong project and that is why my company is the Warrior Woman Project and not just Warrior Woman. Through this book I am going to share with you how to get unstuck, how to understand who you are, how to find ways to love yourself (hopefully more, but for some of you it will be to love yourself), learn that it is okay to be selfish (from the positive meaning of the word) and how to use the 9 Rules to Sort Out Your Shit.

I am Jen Wilson and I am the founder and creator of the Warrior Woman Project.

From this very first chapter I need to request something from you. I want you to take full responsibility for everything you think about while reading this book and every action you take as the consequence of reading it.

Why do I ask you for that sort of commitment?

There are generally 3 types of people who have an opinion around self-help/personal development books / coaching programmes / courses:

1. There are the ones who think it's all juju woo woo nonsense and want no part of it (I have a couple of very close friends in this band) and will probably roll their eyes at you when they see you reading it. If you are not this person, ignore them, this is about you and what works for you. If you are this person, maybe read the book anyway with an open mind.

2. Then there are the ones who buy every book, go on every course, take in all the knowledge and can tell everyone else how to solve their

lives worries but never actually take action on it themselves (I also have a couple of very close friends in this band). If you are this person, I hope that something I say inspires you to make even one change in your life. Let's be honest here; you are looking for something in the reading. If you know someone like this, give them a copy of this book for their collection.

3. The one's who read, listen, learn and take action (I also have a couple of close friends in this band too and I am this person) which is where I hope to inspire you to be, you being the Warrior Woman action taker ready to sort your shit.

I am going to take a stab in the dark that it is unlikely you are not No.1 on that list, unless of course you have picked up the book by accident or been given it as a gift (maybe give it a read through anyway, you never know, you might just enjoy it).

To give you a bit of my background and how this all came about, my story starts on 21st September 2010 with this guy (Brian, now a close friend) who came to talk at my college about a thing called NLP (neurolinguistics programming). NLP is what I discovered to be a life changing way of reprogramming our brains so that we deal with the world in a more positive way and it helps you let go the limiting beliefs that can hold us back from allowing ourselves to be the best version of ourselves. Little did I know when I sat in that class-room listening to some stories that something Brian said would change my life so drastically.

Less than 2 weeks after that day at college I sat down and had a life changing conversation with my husband that would end our marriage and have him move back to Australia (his homeland).

In that conversation, everything that I thought was forever was no more. He was homesick and wanted to move back home to Australia and the reason we had moved back to Scotland was because I was homesick in Australia. There was no way to work round it and I am not the kind of person who would allow someone to make them self unhappy just to make me happy. Life and relationships don't work that way.

My whole life as I thought I knew it was upside down and me, being me, told the world I was 'fine', it was the 'right thing for both of us'. Of course my 'fine' was a lie and I held it together by partying my nights away, and spending my days busy with college work, setting up a business with my friend, working out, eating junk food, having beers for breakfast on the days I didn't need to drive... For about 9 months there was a whole lot of denial, distraction and numbing going on in my world.

My denial that I was anything other than 'fine' came to a breaking point, and then there were tears, and lots of them. I even got fed up with my own crying. My head was all over the place, I just wanted to be alone so I didn't need to talk to anyone, everything was spinning and I couldn't get a thought straight in my head. That was when I started to get some NLP coaching (with Brian) and gradually put my life back together.

This wasn't the first time I had been through a significant change in my life, but it was the first time that I really felt that I needed a helping hand to get through it all. Admitting you need someone to help you and asking for it can feel like a massive challenge in itself, especially if you have always been someone who has managed to sort your head out on your own in the past.

About 18 months before my divorce I went through a career change. After spending 13 years in the travel industry I was no longer inspired or motivated and knew that I needed to do something drastic to change it. Life then felt so difficult, I didn't want to go to work, it was depressing to get up out of bed, some days I really struggled to get through the day without thinking 'is this really all I have to look forward to for the rest of my life?'

There are many stages in life that those questions come up 'have I taken the right path?', 'is this it?', 'am

I missing out on something exciting?', 'am I too old to make changes?' The answer to that last question is no, you are not too old and it's not too late, not until you take your last breath is it too late to make a decision where your happiness is improved.

I didn't know it at the time, but that talk given by Brian in 2010 and the conversation with my now ex-husband was the birth place of the Warrior Woman Project and now the 9 Rules to Sort Your Shit. I realised that I could help other women who like me felt challenged by making changes in their life but know that it is something we just need to do. The challenges I faced not just through my divorce but also the complete change in career at the ripe age of 30 has helped me understand and shape this programme into something that is easy to follow and through my own experience and the clients I have worked with, it is really effective and adaptable to different situations.

Welcome to your journey.

For me the meaning of Warrior Woman comes from my love of the history of the Vikings where the women stood fearlessly on the front line, strong, confident, believing in themselves and fighting for what they believed in. Since then throughout history there have been many female warriors that stood their ground and fought for their lives, happiness and future. The ethos of being a Warrior Woman is about fearlessly taking responsibility for your own life to sort your shit, to make your happiness a high priority, learning to love yourself and to be selfish (in the way the benefits you and everyone else around you), and not watering yourself down to fit in. I am a great believer that if you are just you with all your amazing weirdness, you will attract all the amazing weird people that accept you and fit in your world. Your tribe, your posse, your crew, whatever you want to call it. The rest will gradually move away.

Let me acknowledge this word 'selfish', I can already feel some of you gasping, screwing up your nose or pulling away, but stay with me for a minute so I can explain.

Think of yourself as a glass full of the most delicious drinking water and you share some of that water with your family, friends, boss, partner, neighbour, and the pet. You give, give, give but you don't take any time to go to the tap to refill (you are just too busy with all the give, give, give)... You run out of water, you are thirsty, you get cranky, you snap at people, you can be irrational, you are a moody cow and you make crappy decisions that are generally out of character. Your glass is empty.

This is where your selfish comes in, you learn to stop and refill your glass so you can get a drink too and that way you can keep sharing and keep giving and everyone wins. When you take the time to refill not everyone at first will be happy, especially if you have been a giver up until now. You will even feel a bit guilty at first, but once you take the time, you feel better, the people you give to see you better, then they feel better and everyone is happier and the guilt and expectations will go.

It is the same as when they tell you on the plane to fit your own oxygen mask first... You are no use to anyone if you can't breathe because you die.

So, that is what I mean about learning to be selfish, take a bit of time to refill your glass, look after yourself and not only are you setting a good example to people around you but you are also setting standards of how you need to live to survive happy in your world.

I have been there with the empty glass. I wasn't just a moody cow, I hit total burnout. I kept telling myself that I didn't need any time off because I loved everything that I did (work hard, play hard, you can sleep when you are dead kind of nonsense) and it made me happy doing things for everyone else. What I really was doing was numbing myself from the reality of my marriage ending by keeping so busy there was not time to think or feel. Then I landed on my ass and couldn't get out of bed for nearly 2 weeks. I will go in to more about this in the chapter on self-sabotage.

In the process of recovery from my burnout I had to make a lot of 'selfish' decisions, they weren't easy and it didn't happen overnight. I had to cut ties with people, give up teaching many of my fitness classes and close down 2 businesses that I owned with a friend, take time off, learn to deal with my shit and look after myself better (eating the right foods, and doing the right kind of exercise).

Part of that journey was about taking responsibility for me and my life, it was time for me to realise what I was capable of, stop hiding behind others, set up on my own and work to a new set of rules that I created. I had worked my ass off to gain all these qualifications and now I needed to do something with them. For someone who really didn't like education the first time round, I now have a BSc in Sport and Exercise Science, PGDip Teaching in Further Education (TQFE) qualification and I am an NLP Master Practitioner (among many other qualifications I have gained along the way).

I could only take that step back in to education because I put my happiness first, I realised that I wanted to help people in a much deeper way than booking their holidays. I wanted to make a real impact and difference in the world.

I knew that I needed to help women who like me felt lost and stuck in the world they had worked hard to create throughout their 20's and are now thinking that maybe they want something else, something different, something more. What you have created so far doesn't need to be it for the rest of your life.

I took my time working it out, learned a bit about meditation and the power it has to bring ideas to you, then it came to me when I was lying in bed one day after a morning meditation – I love how stuff like that happens when you are not even thinking about it. It was my unconscious mind working its magic.

I had a vision of the Warrior Woman Project.

I started to write a blog on a daily basis starting to tell my story, make suggestions about different ways to think about the world and deal with life. Within a couple of months my mailing list had more than doubled and I was getting responses from women asking how I knew what was going on in their heads? Was I a mind reader? I had reached in to their hearts and understood exactly where they were and that I knew just the right thing to say at the right time. Then came the online programme and workshops (details can be found over at www.warriorwomanproject.com) and now this book.

The thing is, I was just writing about what I had either been through, was going through or what I could see happening with the women close to me. More recently readers have been reaching out with questions that I anonymously share the question and my answer in the blog.

We are all going through 'stuff', we all have doubts and insecurities and we just need those words, a different point of view or a task that makes us think differently and potentially realise our strengths and capabilities.

Our mission at the Warrior Woman Project is to create a community of women who empower themselves and each other so they live a life that not only makes them happy, but also inspires those around them to do the same. At the Warrior Woman Project, we aim to set an example of self-management, leadership and responsibility not just for our own self but also everyone in the communities we are connected to. We want to create a ripple effect.

The feedback I have had and what I witnessed from these workshops, online programme and one to one coaching sessions has been phenomenal. Changes are happening, confidence is being built, new jobs are being applied for and successfully got, new countries are being lived in and these women are starting to understand how important they actually were and that by being happy in all areas of their life they could actually give more. There is genuine happiness in these women's lives and they are sharing that.

That is not to say that there are not still some struggles and set-backs, we are human and life likes to throw us a curve ball from time to time to remind us that what happens around us is out of our control, but what we do have is control over how we react. Resilience gets stronger all the time to the point where sometimes the curve ball is fun to knock us off balance.

The women working with me through all the different channels are setting a leading example, realising their worth and feeling happier every day. I am not going to bullshit you and tell you they woke up the next day completely changed women, it's hard work and takes effort, they have to face up to new challenges and let go of their shit that they have been using as their security blanket 'it's not my fault' 'poor me'.

They started to take responsibility for their lives, their actions and their own happiness. They stopped waiting for someone else to come and save the day.

With lots of trial and errors, I have now created a structure and formula that works. This formula has now been created as a 12 week online membership programme that you can methodically work through, each week you have access to the next section with instructions, tasks and work to do and implement. You will notice in this book that there are not 12 chapters, the goal setting stage on the course is reviewed twice throughout the 12 weeks and the nutrition programme is completely separate.

Putting it online and writing the blog and this book means I can reach more women globally, more help can be given and the ripple effect keeps going getting bigger and stronger every day. That's not to say that I won't take my workshops outside of Glasgow (I would be delighted to travel with it). My goal is to reach and work with 1 million women through this book, workshops, courses, speeches, and the online membership programme.

The Warrior Woman Project message is simple; you have everything you need within to sort your shit and create the ripple effect. All you need to do is start with you and realise you can only change yourself, lead by example and always do your best.

This leads me in to the very first exercise of the book (yip straight in there in chapter one), it is entirely up to you how you work this, some of you might love to buy a notebook and do everything in the one space, others might prefer to download the resources from www.warriorwomanproject.com/resources and just use those, or make use of the spaces left within the book and others might just want to have a think about it and not actually write anything.

*A note on that, I would strongly advise and encourage you to write out your responses and ideas from each exercise. Not only do you then have a note of this but you also will find it more powerful having written it and created a stronger connection with your thoughts, your mind and your future actions.

Exercise

You will notice that the wheel of happiness doesn't have any headings filled in for you.

I do this because I find that the generic ones although are good, some of the headings can be further broken down or not even relevant to you.

My suggestion is to print off a couple of copies of the wheel, do one general using headings: Personal Development, Relationships, Health, Career/Work, Money, Fun, Family, Spirituality/Religion.

Then any that have more than one meaning or you want to break down further select headings that are most relevant to you. For example let's say that Relationships you score it a 5, some of your relationships might be a 10, some might be a zero – friends, family, romantic, work colleagues, kids are all different relationships. Health could be physical health, mental health, emotional health, fitness, nutrition etc.

Other examples of headings that might be more relevant to you could be:

Relationships (this could be further specified to family, friends, romantic, colleagues), body image, weight, food, religion, spirituality, money, career, personal development, health, social life, attitude, environment (your own living and working space), hobbies, fun, time management, emotional, mental, etc...

If there are other headings or words that resonate better then use them, these are just examples.

0 = despair, you need serious change 10 = delirious, there is nothing that could make it better.

It is useful to date and hold on to your wheel so that you can compare each time you evaluate.

You can get a larger version of the Happiness Wheel at www.warriorwomanproject.com/resources.

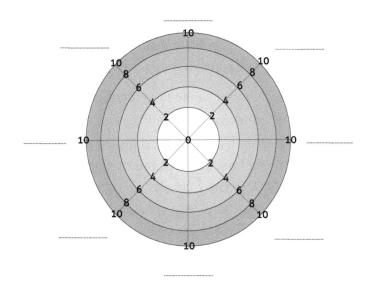

It is also useful to remember that the wheel reflects where you are at in your head at the present time. If you have had a particularly bad week at work or had a fight with a family member then that might be lower than it normally would be.

As much as we are looking for balance in the wheel it would be impossible for us to achieve a 10 in all areas all of the time. If you consider that like the calendar year, our life works in seasons. There will be times that we need to focus more on our careers meaning that our social life might need to be stepped back from a bit. Or there might be a health issue that means you need to be with family more and take a step back from business.

Problems arise when we need to focus on one thing but we prefer to focus on something else (your business needs attention but you are choosing to socialise and procrastinate from the work you need to do). Don't worry if this is happening, we all do it... The important thing here is to recognise that we are doing it and get back on track.

Right now all we are looking for is what is out of balance and checking in with ourselves whether or not it is okay for it to be out of balance right now.

Even writing this book, and forever more, I need to work on myself daily, there are always things that I can do better, bigger challenges to accept, improvements to be made, facing up to things that I want to avoid, but I have come a long way. I believe that we need to leave a legacy and that comes through hard work, living your passions, setting the example, never giving up on ourselves and never settling.

That day back in 2010 I listened, I took action, I made some massive decisions and changes to my life and don't regret a single one. I now run a successful business and through some trials and errors I regularly take time for me to refill my cup so I can work hard, share the love and lead by example.

I hope you enjoy the journey.

Warrior Action

* Accept responsibility for your actions
* Be honest with yourself always
* Breathe
* Give yourself a break

CHAPTER 2

WARRIOR WOMAN RULE #1:
KNOW WHO YOU ARE.

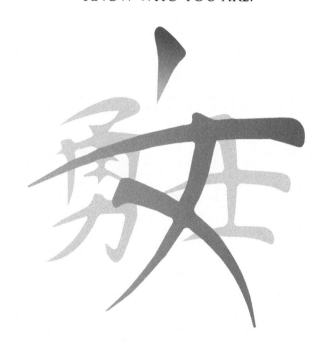

Feeling lost and not sure who you are is a part of growing up – hopefully that is good news for you to know that you are not alone and that at regular points in our life we all go through it. Remember when you started high school? Transitioning through your teen years in to your early 20's when you might have dabbled with different styles, groups of friends, music interests, hobbies etc.

Thinking back we might have seemed more open to trying and testing out new things that we maybe think twice about now that we are 'adulting'... How many arguments did you have with your parents about your hair colour, amount of makeup you were wearing, the length of your skirt or that racket you call music?

As you get older you think that maybe you should feel more settled in life, surely as you grow up you find your 'place' in the world and you shouldn't have to make so many difficult decisions. As a kid you probably couldn't wait to grow up and now as a grown up you probably wish you were still a kid when life was easier. It is at this time as an adult that we are more aware of changes and unsettled feelings going on and maybe we feel less equipped to deal with them, but please be reassured we have the skills to get through what might feel like an overwhelming time and I am going to show you how with these 9 Rules to Sort Your Shit.

It's time to introduce you to Rule #1 and introduce yourself to you.

I think 'just be yourself' has to be worst advice ever given to anyone... How often have you heard the advice 'just be yourself, you are fabulous, people will love you just the way we do', 'you have nothing to worry about' 'if only you could see yourself the way I see you'?

Every single time I heard these statements in the past I was thinking 'yeah, no problem, but... WHO THE HELL AM I???' How can you be yourself when you are not entirely sure who it is you are or what it is you want from life?

'Just take the mask off and expose the real you'. That is another mind blowing statement... Real me?? I didn't know there was a not real me... The thing about masks is we have many of them. We have our work mask, our socialising with work mask, our socialising with friends mask, our spending time with the extended family mask, our first date mask, our dealing with difficult people mask... Basically we have many masks that we can and do wear which depends on the situation that we face.

The problem can arise when we feel really comfortable in one of those masks and use that as our protection to hide behind. If you think of the woman (or maybe you are her) who breaks balls in the boardroom, owning the office floor is where she excels and in every other situation outside of the boardroom she has that same steely approach (except maybe around one or two of her closest friends). Or there is the mum who is there for her kids 24/7 making sure everything is just right for them, making their decisions, getting them organised (she is breaking balls in the family home) and treats all her family and friends in the same way mothering everyone she comes in to contact with.

Maybe you are asking the question 'who do you think I am if I am not the person standing in front of you right now?!'

Every time you are being you, you are being you…

Let me explain. In the car when you are singing your heart out (if you are me, completely out of tune), that is you. When you are in the boardroom kicking ass and controlling the room, that is you. When you are in the supermarket doing your weekly shop, that is also you… Whatever you are doing, it is always a version of you… I am not sure how it would go down if you were in a meeting singing your heart out instead of kicking ass… At the core of all these versions are your values.

It would be fair to say that we have many masks (or hats or labels, whatever you prefer to call them) and each of them has a specific role to help us through the day and fit in to the situation are in at that time.

These masks that we wear from day to day give us some protection and allow us to be adaptable to whatever situation we are dealing with. They allow us to tap in to different parts of our personality and strengths to help us feel like we are winning at life (and they can also hinder us when we feel like we are the furthest thing from winning at life).

So, who the hell are you? Who do you want to be? And what the hell are these values?

Sometimes the masks that can give us protection also can hold us back. Some people might think 'I can't have a career because I am a mum'. 'I don't have time to be a girlfriend I am too busy focusing on my career'. Or 'I'm fat because I'm a chocaholic'... whatever the reason, the excuses are ready.

If you were to overhear someone talking about you, what would you LIKE to hear them say about you? Have a think about it just now, are you that person? Very probably you are at the heart and soul of yourself, but do you let the world see that person so that when they do talk about you, these are the things they say?

Exercise

If you had the choice to be anyone in the world who would you be?

What would you be like?

What would you do?

How would you talk?

How would you dress?

What would your behaviours be like?

What would you achieve in life?

What image do you want to portray to the rest of the world?

What would happen in your world to make you happy every day? Are there people in your world that you would like to be more like?

Part of settling in to yourself is to understand who you want to be so creating a 'To Be' list rather than a 'To Do' list can massively help here. How do you show up 'to be'? That is what that first exercise is about. There is a chance that the mask that you have on just now fills a role that you have maybe fallen in to but hadn't been your life long plan and somewhere along the road you didn't stop to take some time and reassess what and who you want to be going forward.

As a kid maybe you had dreams of exploring the world but after school you went to university then landed a really good job and the opportunity was too good to miss... Or you met the man of your dreams, got married, had kids and really wish you had the opportunity to go to university... Or maybe you went off travelling and are now finding it difficult to 'settle' in to a 'normal' life.

The next part we are going to look at helps you understand what your core values are. These are the character traits that we live by and when we live by the ones that are most important to us decision making is easier, and we feel happier and settled. When you understand your core values it makes it a whole lot easier to learn how to 'just be you' no matter which role you are in.

I remember the first time values were discussed in an NLP coaching session. I looked blankly at Brian thinking 'is this another one of these questions I don't want to answer? Is this going to make me cry?' – It didn't, it cleared a whole lot of stuff up, it was a real lightbulb moment and taking the time to work out my values in life, career and relationships has really helped me work better overall.

I quickly discovered that this was something I NEEDED to know and have been very grateful of ever since, as have all my clients when I have worked through this task with them. I have my lists written out and put in places I see them regularly as a reminder, especially when I am struggling to make a decision, bringing my attention back to the values helps give some clarity.

When things feel like they don't sit right with us, we feel uneasy about decisions that have been made, actions or attitudes from others feel wrong, problems arise, a horrible unsettled feeling can stir up and it is usually when our values are not being met and life is going against your values system.

I had a situation with a company I worked for where the management wanted us (the front line staff) to work for less money, give them more time (unpaid) and supply our own equipment. There was no down line respect or support and we were expected to be the ones doing all the work and bringing in and retaining clients. I very much operate from a helping hand leadership. I only ask of people what I would do myself. My values of respect, trust and connection were being violated and it didn't sit well with me.

One organisation I left, on my last day I was presented with a beautiful gift and parting speech from the customers to thank me for being a great leader and setting the example of caring and respecting everyone in the class. Because I had delivered that, they all repeated those actions with each other. At no time had I ever even considered the example I was setting, I was just doing my job, living by my values. Not a single manager even acknowledged the work I put in or even my departure.

So what are values and how do we work out our own?

Core values are the things that are important to you, not what society thinks you should be (don't confuse morals with values). They are the feelings that whether or not you are aware of it you make your life decisions around. When something feels completely right with you it is because it meets your values, when something doesn't feel right with you it is because it doesn't meet your values. The three main areas but not exclusive that we have values are: career, relationships and life.

Exercise

Working out your values:

You can download a table of example values at www.
warriorwomanproject.com/resources to use - just
remember that list is not exhaustive, there are no right
or wrong answers, you can add or change any of the
words you like. They need to mean something to you.

Sit for a maximum of 3 minutes (time it) and highlight
the ones that jump out at you and make you think, 'yes
that is really important to me'. Write out a list of your
highlighted ones, narrow this down to your top 10 then
put them in order of most to least important.

If you don't want to use the template with the examples, with a blank sheet of paper write down the feelings that are most important to you, once you have a
list of 10-12 words, put them in order of importance.
Don't worry if you get stuck for words, keep thinking,
keep asking yourself 'What else is important to me?'
You might end up with a few words that all have similar meanings, check with yourself if they do mean the
same thing to you or if they are different e.g. Trust and
honesty to some people these are the same, to others
they are completely different. If they are the same, keep
the one that resonates most with you. If they mean
different things and are both important, keep both.

Take the time to do all 3 areas: life, relationships and career. The 3 lists may be very similar (or not at all – remember there is no right and wrong, it's about what works for you), the order of them might be different. For example for some people in their career values security might be really high up on the list of values but in relationships that might be low or non-existent or vice versa.

Tip: write them out on individual post-it notes so you can easily move and change the order or the sheet of paper could get pretty messy, or do it in a word or excel document if you are modern day techy (I like old school paper).

Now you have your list of core values.

Once you have your list, read it, start to understand where these fit in your life and know why they are important to you, look at your life and how it fits round your values. Don't make the values fit round your life. The decisions you make in life are because of these values. When something doesn't feel right it is usually because something is going against a value or values.

Let's have a look at how this might work for you. Say commitment was high on your relationship values and the person you are seeing wants to keep things casual and open. You might first agree to see how it goes, but if it stays that way for a long time and doesn't seem to be moving on to a committed relationship it won't feel good, you won't feel happy about it, you might even start to feel insecure about yourself. That's because the casual arrangement goes against a core value. If the other person doesn't want the commitment, that's not about you being undesirable or not good enough, it's about you having different values that don't match up.

If security is top of your career values being self-employed possibly isn't the right path for you (not saying that there is no security in running your own business, but it's less secure than if you were in a contracted job).

If honesty is up there in any of your lists then a career in politics is likely to be out and any sort of mistruth is going to really piss you off.

Once you start living by your values not only will you be happier but better things will happen, you will feel more settled, and you will feel like you finally understand yourself. Your life will be easier; making decisions will be easier because you understand the 'what and why' of your decision making. The different masks that you wear in your different roles will all have more meaning and understanding and switching between them will be easier. You might find that you don't need to protect yourself so much by hiding in your comfort zone.

Try not to stress about your lists, these are not set in stone and you can change them at any time. The understanding of them should give you peace and freedom in your thinking. Maybe at another time another word will come to your head that will fit better and you can change it. Also as the balance in your life changes the order of them may change too. It is good practice to review and revisit this task maybe every month or two or if you feel like the world isn't fitting to see if things have changed. As your life situations change, and as you grow as a person, your values may shift around a bit too.

This task is about helping you learn and understand how to be the real deal so you can indeed 'just be yourself' no matter which mask/hat you are wearing.

Now that you have a better understanding of yourself, you may now find that it can also help you understand people around you better. If there are people that you clash with all the time, it could be that your values are not aligned and by understanding this allows you to adapt and manage them better – you can't expect the other person to adapt if they are not in a place of working on themselves or interested in being adaptable. You could always give them the gift of this book but in the meantime you are taking responsibility for being adaptable now that you have the better understanding.

Warrior Action

* Work out your values for life, career & relationships

* Know and understand your values (have them written in a diary or somewhere you can easily access them)

* Be aware of other people's values when there is a conflict and understand where they are coming from

* Review them regularly to make sure that they are still relevant

* Do what feels right for you, not what you think other people expect of you

* Give yourself a break

* Breathe

CHAPTER 3
WARRIOR WOMAN RULE #2:
DREAMS & GOALS, KNOW WHAT YOU WANT

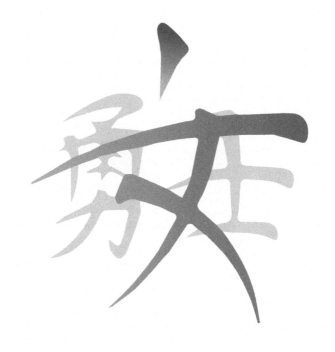

I spent a lot of time through my school years day dreaming (I am a Pisces). I was uninspired and disengaged for most of school life. There were a couple of teachers that sparked my interest, my 1st year art teacher Miss Wilson and 1st year history and modern studies teacher Mr Snee. I don't know what it was about them or those classes but I did well in them, I paid attention and got good marks... Unfortunately that was the only year I had either of them and after that I would sit down in class then check out, dreaming about what life would be like when I was a grown up and could make my own decisions.

The first thing I did when I walked out the school gates on that last day was chuck all my books in the bin...

I was going to college to study travel and tourism and then get to see the world...

Much to my surprise I did really well at college, in fact, I got student of the year! I asked the senior lecturer if she was sure she had the right person when she phoned to tell me. I had never been top of the class never mind top of 60 college students! That first award or recognition made me realise that just maybe I could in fact do more with my life and that my school years were not the big set up for life that they had been made out to be. Many people say your school years are the best years of your life and that makes me sad. That makes me think that they have stopped living, stopped dreaming, and stopped believing there is more to this life.

The purpose of life is to live a happy life.

Our dreams are what we hope for to fulfil that purpose, we set goals to help us fulfil those hopes and dreams and I don't want to burst your bubble but, we are going to fail at parts along the way. Sometimes those failures will be small bumps in the road (how do you find the cash to travel the world?) or they can be a fork in the road where you have to decide one way or the other (do we stay married or go our separate ways?) or they can seem like unclimbable mountains (I don't have the skills, knowledge, time or faintest idea where to start my own business). The important thing to remember is you need step up, understand what is important to you (those values from the last chapter), think about how else could work, what was it that didn't work before and try something else and think about reaching out for help.

When you get the conditions right you will succeed and very few of us, very few times will get it right first time (that is good news). It is only as we get older that we seem to have a problem with failing at things. Watch a baby, see how many times they try something and fail and try again...Would you ever let that baby give up trying to walk? Failing is how we grow and develop. At no point does anyone ever tell the baby to stop trying, they have tried enough... Try again, and again, and again, always encouraging them. At that age embarrassment of failure isn't something we are even aware of existing, we learn that a few years later and then most of us let it hold us back.

The important thing to work out if you don't instinctively know is what your dreams are, why it is you have them, how to set the goals and create the plan to get you on the road to success and failure.

I saw Colonel Chris Hadfield speak in Edinburgh, his tour was called *The Sky is Not the Limit*... I love that title.

The stand out point for me and it was something that I had never heard anyone else say, was that it really doesn't matter if you never achieve the dream but if you do everything you can to work towards that dream you won't ever live a life disappointed.

This was a revolutionary and profound moment for me... 'it doesn't matter if you never achieve that dream' Who knew?! Permission had just been granted to dream even bigger than I imagined possible and it be okay if I didn't get there... If you are following the path to the dream then you are always going to be doing things for a reason, they will usually be things that you enjoy – I am not sure when I was sitting for hours writing essays for uni I would have said I was enjoying it but I always knew there was a purpose to the action and that makes the difference.

One of the many amazing and successful women I know runs dance schools for kids and had posted one day about the success of her business and how a teacher at school had told her dance wasn't a real job and she should do something real... Thankfully she ignored that teacher, followed her dream and is reaping the success of her hard work.

There will always be people who will encourage you to give up on your dreams or tell you that what you want is out of reach... Maybe they gave up on their dream, maybe they believed someone when that was what they were told... Does that give them the right to tell you that you can't or shouldn't chase your dreams? This is your life, and your responsibility.

How much happier will you be if you are doing everything you can to be the person you want to be?

If you want to be a top surgeon then you need to go to medical school and work your way through the ranks, departments, courses, shadowing other top surgeons. There is no point settling for a course in accounting because that is your best subject at school.

If you want to be a movie star you need to get in front of the camera, get those parts as extras, go to the auditions, put yourself in situations where you might get your break, anything else is a stop gap to give you money until you get your break.

To be successful you need to create the right conditions to make the results happen. To create the right conditions you need to set some goals and to get those results you need to understand why they are important to you.

Start at the top, what is the big picture? What is the dream? If your life was picture perfect, what would that look like? Be honest, this is your dream. Then work your way back, breaking things down in to smaller steps and goals always with that dream in mind. Strip each step back, breaking it down until you get to a To Do list that doesn't terrify the life out of you. This can be the route plan to get you moving towards the dream.

In the first chapter we looked at your Wheel of Happiness to see where we are in life, what is out of balance? How does that make you feel right now? Let's just say your decided one of your headings was romantic relationships and that was down at a 3 or 4, maybe that is okay for you because being in a romantic relationship is not a high priority to you right now... But maybe part of your dream is to be happily married with children, then this is going to change the priority of how and when you make this a focus in your life.

Not everyone will be a daydreamer like me; in fact, it's much more common for my clients to have a really blank expression on their faces when I ask them what the dream is, and what it is they really want? There is often a mix of 'I don't know', 'I haven't really thought about it' or shyness about saying out loud what it is they want because they don't want to come across as selfish, egotistical or mad. Chris Hadfield was 9 when he knew he wanted to be an astronaut even though they had never at that time sent a Canadian in to space, his whole education and career was focused on taking the necessary courses and steps to give him the right education and skills just in case the time came that he could be sent up to space. His dreams came true; he was 33 before he became actively involved in the space programme and 42 before he actually got in to space.

Someone is going to be an astronaut, a prime minister, president, Royal Princess, head teacher, top surgeon, supermodel, multi-million pound bra designer, award winning actor, bestselling author, owner of the Virgin brand, Olympian... Why can that someone not be you? Regular people do extraordinary things all the time. So many people that we highly respect at the top of industries have at one time been a 'normal' person just like us, living life, making decisions, working with the road that they have been set on. Reading autobiographies is a real eye-opener to the struggles and journeys many at the top have been through.

So, what do we do when we have no idea what the dream is?

Please don't worry if you are sitting there thinking 'Oh Jen, I have no idea what I want to do'. Think back to when you were a kid, before 'the real world' killed your imagination; what did you love to do? What sparks your interest? What can you get lost for hours doing? Are you just scared to say it out loud? – don't worry, this is a book, I can't hear you.

Maybe you genuinely don't have a 'dream' and that is totally okay, maybe you have lots of things that you are curious about. Follow those curiosities, read, learn, explore, dive in to the possibilities that they create. Maybe a 'dream' will come to you at some other time. In the meantime don't stress about it, don't settle for what you have and don't give up on yourself.

Tip: Meditate – most of my best ideas come to me during or after meditation. Before you break in to a panic about not being able to meditate, I have been there, I have read the books, listened to the apps, been on the courses. The best advice I got was to just focus on your breath. Even if it is for 2 breaths, your mind wanders then you bring it back focus on 2 breaths, your mind wanders. That is better than not trying or declaring meditation isn't for you. It doesn't need to be for long, a few minutes every day will calm and quiet your mind.

Download an app with guided meditation or sit and breathe and just think about your breathing. Thoughts will sneak in to your head, and you will drift off lost in your thoughts, all you need to do is be aware of them and take your focus back to your breath.

If sitting still to breathe isn't your thing then if you can get out for a walk and focus on your breathing there (leave your phone behind, no technology to distract you), fresh air and focused breathing will really clear your head.

A lot of this is about taking away the distractions of life, letting your brain settle so you can let your thoughts in.

If nothing comes through to you during your meditation (or quiet time), keep doing it anyway, it's good for your mind. Take your time, and look for the things that make you feel curious, what do you want to know more about? What sparks an interest? I like to look for inspiration on things like Pinterest, there are some fantastic vision boards on there (be warned though, you will lose hours of your day when you enter in to that minefield of pretty images). Start to create your own pin boards or if you don't want to be stuck on your phone, create a real life vision board. From magazines, newspapers etc. collect images that inspire you. Maybe it is your dream house, car, job, outfit, travel destinations... It is your board, put on it whatever you like.

Once you start to create an image of what you would like, whether its travel, career, relationships, health, interests, hobbies, general life improvements it can make the whole goal setting, planning process easier.

If you like to journal, you can review your plan every single day, I have friends that spend time focusing on their vision daily. My week isn't that structured and I find it difficult to review daily, so I review these every 4 weeks (or the 1st of every month). Whatever the frequency, make sure that it works for you and not only are you on track to achieving your goals but also to make sure they are still the goals you want to achieve.

Have you ever applied for a job only to realise at the interview process that it's not actually the right job for you? Or you start on a weight loss journey only to realise that eating cake every now and again is more important because it is part of your social life and that eating salad and vegetable sticks every day or counting points or sins sucks and you are missing out on a lifestyle that you actually enjoyed. Having curves is not the end of the world, if you love your ass that is way more important (more on that later in the book). Or, have you joined a gym to realise that you hate being stuck indoors all the time and that structured exercise is not for you?

It's important to understand that just because you said you were going to go one way, it is ok to change your mind when you realise that what you thought would make you happy actually doesn't. Nothing is set in stone; the outcome of any goal should ultimately be to make you happy in the long term.

**Note here, sometimes some of the journey is tough, studying, training, portion control etc. can be a pain in the ass but we have to sometimes make short term sacrifices to gain long term happiness. Always keep your end goal in sight to remind you why you are doing what you are doing, particularly when it feels like a struggle. The struggle is real and it is part of your journey making you stronger.

Once you figure out what it is you want, you then need to work out how you are going to get it. Some of the questions you will want to consider:

* What do you need to do?
* What are you prepared to sacrifice?
* Who can you get to help you?
* What are the financial costs? What are the emotional costs?
* Who else does it affect?

You also need to consider a contingency plan. There will be times when you are all set to go and something gets in your way – the kids get sick, your boss or a client calls an unexpected emergency meeting, you don't get on to the course you want to get on... Plans then will need to change, but rather than giving up you need to do the best you can in the circumstances. Take a moment to consider 'what is the best way to deal with this situation?'

It is up to you to set your conditions in place to allow everything to come together. Call in help, get extensions on deadlines, and identify other routes that you can take.

You need to put yourself in to the right mind-set, focus on the outcome and make sure that changes out of your control don't allow you to self-sabotage (self-sabotage being when you put obstacles in your own way and give yourself excuses to get out of things e.g. the kids, the boss, clients, the weather etc.). Don't worry we go in to this in detail in the next chapter. .

For example:

You have packed your gym stuff, set the alarm, and prepared all your food ready to go first thing in the morning.

The alarm went off, you can hear the rain battering off the windows, and you didn't get the best sleep so decide that you are cosy in bed, so you won't get up for the gym but plan to go at the end of the day instead.

You get up later, then during the day nothing seems to go to plan, one of your friends calls and invites you to the pub after work.

You have 2 options here...

1. You can ditch the gym and head to the pub 'for one', you can start fresh tomorrow when you promise yourself you will get up and go to the gym.

Or

2. You can thank your friend for the invite but you made a promise to yourself that the extra hour in bed was a compromise for a post work gym session. You can always invite your friend along to the gym.

Obviously option 2 is the one that will keep you closer to your goal than option 1.

Life is full of temptations that take us off in other directions, sometimes these other occasional distractions are okay but the problem arises when it happens a lot. How often do you let that happen to you? I'll start tomorrow / on Monday / when I get paid / when the kids are in bed... They are all excuses that delay your start and your potential success.

When something gets in the way, stick as close to the original plan as you can. Be prepared to let go then reconnect when you can and as best you can don't let it stress you or upset you. I used to get really upset when people expected me to go along to things that interfered with my gym time (I was in the gym 5 or 6 days a week so the occasional missed session wasn't going to do me any harm, more likely it was doing me good). Once you get yourself on a roll it is good to keep going and I know that some people if they fall out of routine even for one day it can knock them off for weeks. Acknowledge if that is the type of person you are and prepare to be strict with yourself to get back on track as soon as possible (or get a coach to hold you accountable).

As humans we are conditioned to desire and seek familiarity, the unpredicted and unknown can make us feel uneasy. The feeling of being overwhelmed can be numbing, we can feel dizzy, breathless, foggy headed, fearful - the fear can be paralyzing and can leave you feeling prepared to settle with what you have rather than chase the dream. It can even have you feeling uncertain of what your dream actually is. This often happens when we are trying to deal with and take on too many things or we start taking on other peoples 'stuff' to use as a distraction and excuse that we have no time for ourselves.

If we get to this point it is important to stop and take a breath, take a step back from as much as possible to assess the situation in front of us (working with a coach is a really good idea if this is how you are feeling, they will know the right questions to ask). To be able to do this is an act of bravery. You are standing up for yourself. Being brave and consistently taking steps in the direction of your dream is the key to success here. It doesn't matter how small the step is, it's better than no step. We admire people who are resilient and keep pushing forward... Be that person you admire.

I set a goal of writing this book, the first draft I sat in an internet café every Saturday for hours working, making progress, fighting with my laptop as I seem to get viruses uploaded on what felt like a daily basis and the flash pen didn't always save my work even though I religiously hit that save icon.

The second draft I got a notebook and wrote most of it by hand before typing it up. I originally started out working with a publisher and then changed direction to self-publish after the second draft had been reviewed. We had a conversation and they said that they didn't think I would like the changes they wanted to make to it because they wanted to 'water my voice down' (what you will learn if it hasn't been obvious already, the Warrior Woman Project is about being you and not watering yourself down to fit in).

I missed many beautiful days in the sun; I had to postpone plans and spent a fortune on tea to achieve this goal... If you are reading this book now, it means I was successful, eventually, even if it took about a year longer than originally planned. I reached out, got help and succeeded.

To get the things we want in life not only do we need to be prepared to fail, but also be prepared to prioritise, compromise and miss out on some things to get something better.

Goal + Plan + Contingency + Determination = Success/ Dream

Exercise:

You can download your Dream, Goal, Plan worksheet from www.warriorwomanproject.com/resources.

Have your Wheel of Happiness from Chapter 1 and your values from Chapter 2 will help you too. From these you are going to work out your goals for the next month.

If you use your phone or an online calendar, set monthly reminders to review the wheel and goals to see where you are, if you are on track and if you are still moving in the right direction. If you use a manual calendar, get writing in it now to plan out to the end of the year in it a reminder to review. Whichever calendar you are using, schedule in the time and stick to it.

Warrior Action

* Meditate

* Know or at least have an idea of what the big dream is

* If you can't think of a dream, follow your curiosities

* Do the things that make you happy

* Write out your dreams, this can be in a journal or on a vision board, whatever works best for you

* Never let anyone tell you your dream is ridiculous – it's your dream, not theirs

* Write out your goals

* Create a plan and a To Do list and action something on it every single day

* Even the smallest step is still a step

* Give yourself a break

* Breathe

CHAPTER 4
WARRIOR WOMAN RULE #3: QUIT WITH THE EXCUSES

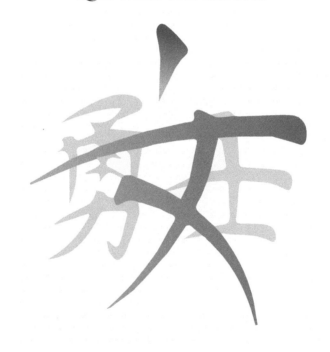

In chapter 3 I briefly mentioned the term self-sabotage. This is something many of us seem to have mastered quite successfully, yet it is the thing that stops us from being a true Warrior Woman, it holds us back from chasing our dreams and finding true peace within ourselves. It's the excuses we use to not achieving what we say we want.

Probably the easiest way to explain self-sabotaging is with our diets because nearly every woman I have worked with struggles in this area even if they don't struggle with their weight. Whether it is a new year's resolution, another Monday is rolling round, you have a holiday coming up, a wedding or are just generally feeling crap about the way you look or feel we frequently self-sabotage...

We have a grand plan that we are going to eat healthy all week because we want to feel good. We either don't make the time to get organised or buy in all the ingredients and supplies that we need. We are all set to go, lunches are made, breakfast is prepared the night before, we know what is for dinner, and we have our snacks all planned out...

Then someone suggests going out for lunch. It's been a shitty morning and what you have planned is just not as appealing as the local pub lunch...

Now going to the pub for lunch doesn't mean it's all going to fail. We can still eat well by carefully selecting the healthier option from the menu but the macaroni cheese and chips is calling out to comfort you so you go for that. That was sabotage number 1. Then at about 3pm you hit a slump as the heavy lunch makes you feel sluggish so you have a coffee and a couple of biscuits to get you through the afternoon. There is sabotage number 2. Then later you are exhausted, the thought of making dinner is just too much and you have ruined your diet today anyway so you sit down with a glass of wine and a bag of crisps or some crackers and cheese thinking what's the point, you can start fresh tomorrow. And that is sabotage number 3...

At any point through that day you had choices to make, often, instead of thinking further ahead and keeping a goal in mind we react to the instant situation. If we are stressed, sad, bored, angry or don't want to see boring we make rash decisions with an 'I don't care' attitude.

This doesn't just happen with our eating; it can be the job you want that you look for where you wouldn't be selected for the post instead of focusing on your strengths and how you can fit it in. Making time for yourself but you never have time, if your best friend calls in a crisis everything is dropped and you make time for them...

It is so much easier when it's not your fault... Bad news for you... It is your fault. You are the one in control of the decisions you make and the support you reach out for. It

You say you want to be better so you need to stop giving yourself excuses. You say you want to look better so that you will feel better about yourself, so that you will feel more confident, happier. You say you want to find love but it seems you don't even love yourself...

* Have a think about these questions:
* Do you ever prioritise yourself?
* Do you make snap decisions without thinking about your end goal?
* Do you eat for health?
* Do you exercise or do activities that keep you healthy and make you happy?
* Do you have hobbies, interests that entertain you?
* Are you learning new things every day to develop yourself in to an even more amazing person?

If the honest answer to any of these questions is no (and that includes answers of hesitation, sometimes or not really) then you need to ask yourself why? If you have taken time through the previous chapters to work out who you are, and thought about your dreams and goals, then you want to keep these at the front of your mind, stop telling yourself it is okay, you will start tomorrow or whatever your excuse is.

'I'm not worth it', 'I don't deserve this' 'I'm not good enough' are just a few of the things you might be telling yourself.

We might not say these out loud, or to anyone else but we sure as hell are thinking and saying them to ourselves inside and we need to stop. I know this because I have been guilty of this too and I still need to pull myself in to check at times. For some reason it feels easier to be down on yourself than saying 'you are worth more than this, you can do this, you are awesome'.

Having these constant doubts and excuses are what holds us back from success, holds us back from happiness and of course cushions us from failure. Brené Brown discusses this in her Power of Vulnerability book, it is easier to prepare yourself for disappointment so it doesn't feel as bad when it happens, but then the problem with this is we miss out on feeling joy. It isn't possible to just numb the negative emotions, when we switch off the negative, we also switch off the positive ones too - this is not good, but what is good news is the more we experience bad or negative emotions, the better we get at dealing with them as we become more resilient and realise that sometimes shit things just happen and we can get up and move on.

This then brings me on to thinking about how we speak to ourselves. Have you ever stopped to take notice of that voice inside your head? I would put money on the fact that (unless you have done work on this before) quite often she is not very nice to you. She puts you down, ridicules you, and creates self-doubt. I used to refer to mine as the 'sergeant major' until I demoted her. When I was at the gym to get me moving more or lifting heavier I would call myself a 'fat, lazy bitch' to motivate myself.

When you think about the things you say to yourself, do you ever speak like that to any of your friends? Or had a friend speak to you like that? My money would be on no, and if you have friends that speak to you like that I want you to think about why you are friends with them? If it is to keep you in your place I would ask you to consider not spending much time with those 'friends' anymore. So why do you speak to yourself like that and let yourself away with it?

If you are reading that last part thinking, 'Jen, I know that I am good enough and deserve the best, I speak to myself in a positive way...' If you are already achieving everything that you want to achieve, you look and feel amazing and are delighted with what you see when you look in the mirror – your external appearance as well as your internal self then fantastic, keep doing what you are doing, you are there, you are a Warrior Woman and self-sabotage isn't something you need to worry about.

For the rest of us...

Other than that voice inside your head, there might be people around you questioning you, doubting your abilities. My question to you is, why do you keep them around? Why are you letting them feed your own self-doubt and self-sabotage?

We want to be around people who have a positive energy that inspires and motivates us and makes us want to be better people and believe in us particularly when we are struggling to believe in ourselves.

Where possible we want to spend less time with people who bring us down, drain our energy and validate your self-sabotage. Probably the most common reason for others to try to pull us back is because if you are doing well and are happy then they feel guilty that they are not taking action themselves.

It is not just our emotional health you need to consider, another thing that you should be considering is our physical health.

* How is your skin looking?
* Are your eyes bright and sparkling?
* Is your hair strong and shiny?
* Are your nails and nail beds looking healthy?

When you have things like skin breakouts and conditions (like eczema and psoriasis), dull eyes, bloodshot eyes, and your hair and weak nails are all tell-tale signs that you are not really looking after ourselves well. You need to look at what you are eating and if you are drinking enough of and the right kind of fluids, but also you need to be considering how much stress you are under and the quality of your sleep.

When you look in the mirror, are you a shape and size you are happy with?

How are your moods from day to day, even morning to evening?

What about your energy levels and motivation?

Again, all of these can be signs that we are doing things on a daily basis that suggest we are not taking care of ourselves (inside and out). It is daily self-sabotage at its base level when we don't eat the right foods, get enough sleep, and/or deal with stress in a way that is beneficial to us.

If this is the case I would like to bring you back to questions such as:

* Why are you not taking better care of your-self?

* What is so important that your health and wellbeing is not a priority?

* Why is it when you start working towards a goal, reach a level of success you hit a wall and stop?

* Why do you not just keep going, get to the wall and climb over?

* What is it that makes you think this is it; this is the best I can have?

Tiredness and stress have a big effect on decision making and can be the root cause of some self-sabotaging behaviours. How often do you make crap food choices because you can't be bothered or, you are having a shit day or, everyone else is eating cake/drinking wine?

So, we have addressed the many different levels and streams of self-sabotage, just because there is a label for it does not mean that it's okay. But, now we know what it is we have something to work with.

The thing with this self-sabotage (or any belief about yourself) is when you believe that it's something that you do, then you are more inclined to use it as the excuse (sometimes even without realising you are). In your head you run the line 'I self-sabotage everything I do, that's just me' – here you are giving yourself a label just like the labels we talked about in chapter 2, you are not your label. This is a behaviour that you do rather than something that you are... Think of that as the Law of Attraction the wrong way round, instead of putting out positive hopes and desires to get positive back, you are putting out negative decisions and excuses that brings back negative actions and situations.

So how do we regain control and start moving in the right direction? A way to get past this and reverse this negative law of attraction is to first recognise when you are self-sabotaging, this means looking out for patterns in your behaviour and results. If you want to change the pattern then we get to break the habit. Self-sabotage can feel like a brick wall that we hit, when you find the wall, climb it, dig through it, get round it, make it crumble, beat it. Don't let it beat you.

To help you break the pattern, work through the questions in this next exercise. You need to answer the questions honestly, you are the only one that knows this stuff and by understanding where you are coming from and what you allow to get in your way allows you to break your habits.

Exercise:

What is it that stops you from sticking with your goal?

What is it you believe about yourself that stops you from staying on track? (what doubts about yourself do you have?)

What is it about the action that you don't want to do? (Is there a particular part that you don't want to do?)

Why is it okay to not stick to the plan?

Where is that coming from? What is that voice inside your head telling you?

Why do you think this challenge you are avoiding can't take you to a place of better happiness?

If you have success what does that mean to you? How will things be different / better for you?

These questions should help you identify what it is that is holding you back. When you have a better under-standing of what it is that holds you back you can then ask yourself 3 simple questions;

* COULD I let this feeling go?

* WOULD I let this go?

* WHEN will I let this go?

Go back and look at your values list from Chapter 2. When you apply them to why you want to achieve your goals it can make it easier to stop giving yourself excuses.

If you are resisting this exercise then we can look at it from a different angle...

* Where will you be in 6 months if you keep self-sabotaging? Look back over the last 6 months to get an idea –are you heavier? Even less fit? Still in the same job? Unhappier?

* How often at the end of the day do you wish you had just got up and gone to the gym in the morning?

* How demotivated do you feel when you put your work clothes on and they feel a bit tighter instead of looser?

* How much more fun would it be playing with the kids if you feel energised and not stressed, exhausted and run down?

* How do you feel on your commute to work to that job that you absolutely hate?

* How much better would it be if that was your trigger that stopped you and said:

* F*ck this, I don't want to feel like crap today / tomorrow / anymore? I want to feel the best I can all day every day.

* I want to look good & feel good. I don't want to hate myself anymore...

* How pissed off with yourself do you need to get before you take action?

* 'I will when I am ready...'

* How do you know when you are ready?

* What is it you are going to be ready for?

"It's a terrible thing, I think, in life to wait until you're ready. I have this feeling now that actually no one is ever ready to do anything. There is almost no such thing as ready. There is only now. And you may as well do it now. Generally speaking, now is as good a time as any." *Dr House (Hugh Laurie)* – How good was that TV show?!

Why do you need to be ready? Why is it you feel that you need to be ready for something? Will you ever be ready? Or are you using it as an excuse to stall because you are afraid? This chapter is really full of thought provoking questions, all of them are useful for you to consider and acknowledge the answers so you can progress.

Image how it will feel to be sitting with a friend enjoying a coffee and cake guilt free rather than inhaling it down with your head in the fridge door so no one sees you? Or how much better it will be when you say no to invitations to things you don't want to go to because you have committed yourself to doing something that you do want to do for you...

Someone once told me that to be successful you have to be in a risk taking mind-set, to be in a risk taking mind-set you need to not be in a self-sabotage mind-set. You need to be prepared to do something different to get a positive change.

So, risks... I don't really like that word, let's call them little challenges or obstacles ... risk sounds a bit scary, I mean risk assessments are looking for danger and we are not looking for danger. We are looking for those little challenges/obstacles that in our head seem a bit uncomfortable, maybe unfamiliar, but if we think back to all the other little challenges/obstacles we have overcome in life and turned out well (or not as bad as we imagined)... Those are the 'risks' we want to take to help us overcome our self-sabotage.

I am all too familiar with what goes on in our heads when we start thinking about the little challenge/obstacle. Our imagination takes control, every 'what if' scenario runs through our head and before we know it there is a complete catastrophic soap opera running in our head. This is not real, this is our imagination (usually fuelled by the TV, social media and movies that we watch).

Let's take a step back for a moment and look at this from a different angle.

* What is the real situation that you are facing?
* If this situation was your friend's situation, what would you tell them to do?
* How would you reassure them that they will be okay?
* What advice would you give them to move forward?

Example 1

Our Mission: To look and feel great in our summer dress and swimwear on holiday

Our Plan: To eat really well, get to the gym every day.

Our Self-Sabotage: 'I have been good all week and I deserve a treat' – that treat can end up being a whole weekend binge because the weeks 'being really good' was way too restricting but it's okay, I will start again on Monday. Or something upsetting or stressful happens and you need to numb the pain with all your comfort foods.

Risk: Understand that the 'go hard or go home' 'all or nothing' methods are a set up to fail. Too much restriction cannot be sustained and you will make yourself even less happy than before, especially if you feel deprived. Accept small sustainable lifestyle changes which will mean slower results but you will be able to maintain them. The biggest risk here is acceptance of the beautiful being that you are right now and that change can't happen overnight.

Example 2

Our Mission: To be in a happy, perfect, secure relationship with our ideal mate.

Our Plan: To have him/her spot us somewhere, approach us, sweep us off our feet, declare undying love for us and live happily ever after.

Our Self-Sabotage: Waiting for someone else to approach us, why do they need to be the ones to show all the vulnerability? Or set up an online dating profile, date everyone and anyone that asks then accept the one that sticks around even when they are not the right one for you. Or be so guarded that you deflect anyone who dares look at you while declaring that there is no one out there and poor you is going to be alone forever so you might as well get the cats in now.

Risk: Firstly falling in love with yourself, and every part of you flaws and all. This will become easier when you have your values lists and know who you are and what you want and need to allow values with another to fall in line (this doesn't mean that they need to have an exact match list but they need to compliment and balance each other). Be prepared to put yourself out there and potentially be rejected with the caveat that if you know and understand your values rejection isn't really rejection, it is a misalignment of values. The biggest risk here is accepting and loving yourself first, without that there won't be a match.

These are just a few examples where initially you think the risk is going to be pretty big, but when you step back and break it down it is not as overwhelming as you first thought.

So, stop beating yourself up just because you have made mistakes in the past, just because you are not exactly where you would like to be in your life. You are worth the effort, you do deserve it and you are good enough. Live in the moment – not in the past because it's gone and can't be changed and the future, it's still to happen, and it can be however you want it to be.

It's time for to fall in love with yourself, show yourself some respect and start trusting yourself to give things a go.

There comes a time in every Warrior Woman's life that she stops bullshitting herself. She gets pissed off with herself and realises it is time to take responsibility, control and make herself a priority, at the end of the day it is down to her to make the change and be happy.

Exercise

Write a list of the 5 things you hate about yourself.

Then write a list of the 5 things love or are most happy with.

Using the 5 things you are most happy with, look at how you can use them to your advantage, to change the things you are least happy with?

Write it down. Make a plan. Start working on it. The time to stop self-sabotaging is over.

Warrior Action

* Do the exercises in this chapter
* Answer the questions honestly
* Be around the right people
* Find a mentor(s) or coach(es) for all areas of your life, these don't necessarily need to cost money although in some areas of expertise it may be worth it. They can be a boss, someone in another department that has skills you want to learn, a good friend that you respect and admire or a friend of a friend.
* Call yourself out and analyse the risk (the real risk)
* Start with small risks that you know are not the end of the world either way to build some confidence and reassure you that your world won't end if things don't work out how you hope.
* Give yourself a break
* Breathe

CHAPTER 5
WARRIOR RULE #4
BREATHE, STOP AND BREATHE

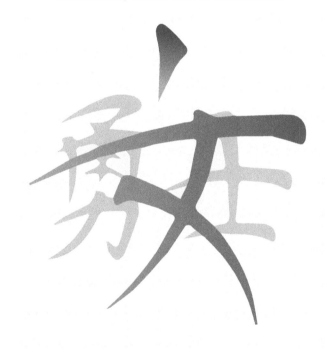

All this talk of self-sabotage and risk taking (or avoid-ance of risk taking) brings us to the lovely world of stress.

The dictionary definition of stress:

Noun – a state of mental or emotional strain or tension resulting from adverse or demanding circumstances.

Verb – cause mental or emotional strain or tension

I am usually someone who doesn't really let things bother me, My mood is neither up nor down when faced with challenges and I pretty much take things in my stride...

What I discovered in the years post my divorce that I was someone who did not deal with emotional stress very well, up until that point in my life the only real emotional stress I had had to deal with was death of a couple of family members, I was lacking in emotional intelligence.

I had always been referred to as a 'strong person' who could deal with anything and at that point I felt that is who and what I was expected to be and rolled with it.

What I realised I was very good at was numbing my emotions. I had regular conversations that I wasn't bothered, it was the right thing to happen for both of us (which it was), or that I was too busy to be worrying about it – a busy mind doesn't have time to be sad.

My head was firmly buried in the sand and I was numbing my pain with busyness, food, drink and 'fun'. I could not be alone and I could not be idle – now I realise these should have been really loud alarm bells ringing and they probably were I just chose not to hear them. I managed to ignore and numb the pain for about 18 months before I started to deal with things (I started going for NLP therapy).

It wasn't until early 2013 that the stress (that I had been burying) bit me on the ass and completely floored me. I was completely out of action for 2 full weeks (getting out of bed to get to the bathroom took all my effort) and it took nearly another 18 months for me to fully recover. Had the doctor's not scared the shit out of me mentioning the possibility of cancer like symptoms I would have possibly ignored them and gone back to my old ways and ended up a whole lot worse off.

Stress can be your best friend at times and also your worst enemy. We need the stress responses for survival… Way back in the day it saved us from being eaten by wild animals. These days though, the wild animal that is killing us comes in the form of our hectic

24/7 lifestyles, overworking and not taking enough care of ourselves and our wellbeing.

I read a lot and an interesting finding about sleep deprivation was that only 2 consecutive nights of less than 7 hours sleep is considered sleep deprivation (how many hours a night do you get??) and there is a growing thinking that this can be linked to some illnesses including obesity, cancer, depression, and anxiety among others. Sleep deprivation is probably one of the most common stresses that the clients I have worked with have, for some it is getting to sleep, others being restless or not staying asleep all night and others waking up really early.

Common symptoms of stress (this list is not exhaustive):

* Anxiety,
* Depression
* Overwhelm
* Confusion
* Panic (including attacks)
* Lack of ability to chill out
* Burnout (losing your mojo)
* Low or no libido
* Constant unexplained headaches
* Nausea

* Binge eating /no appetite
* Skin break outs such as eczema acne and psoriasis
* Bad sleeping patterns (not sleeping enough, too much or at sporadic times)
* Muscle tension (how is your back, neck and shoulders?)
* Mood swings or a bad temper

**Please know that some of these symptoms may be related to an underlying illness or side effects to medication (including the contraceptive pill) or connected to your monthly cycle so always get checked out by a health professional and track your moods and feelings for a couple of months to see if there is any pattern developing.

I imagine many of us have experienced at least one or two of those symptoms in our lifetime, sometimes relating to stress even if we haven't particularly identified the link, sometimes it has been an illness which may (or may not) have been brought on by stress which is believed to weaken the immune system.

Some of the more common causes of stress I have come across with myself and my clients (again this list is not exhaustive, what is stressful to one person could be complete chill out to another):

* Working too much, not taking time to relax
* Not breathing properly (slow deep breaths are ideal to reduce stress)
* Not sleeping well – even getting 7-8 hours per night and waking up tired
* Not taking time to play / be creative
* Too much exercise
* Drinking stimulants (coffee, energy drinks, alcohol)
* Overthinking or not letting things go.

With some of the symptoms it can be 'which came first the chicken or the egg' for example, I suffer from eczema; I have done since I was 18 months old. Sometimes a breakout will be caused by food intolerance (usually dairy, wheat, sugar) but sometimes I could eat those things and not have a breakout... There would also be times when my diet was angelic and I would get a breakout...

It drove me mad until I went on a yoga breathing course where we spent 3 hours learning how to breathe properly (you would be surprised how many different ways of breathing there is). On the day of the course I had an eczema breakout, the following morning I woke up and my skin was pretty much clear. Any time I start to get a breakout now I take some time out and focus on my breathing and the symptoms reduce.

As I said before, I am not a health care professional who can prescribe treatments, but this works for me for this specific stress. When I focus on my breathing it reduces stress in my body reducing the symptoms. My thought process of 'if I breathe properly I can have bread' is quite the motivation.

You will have noticed in the Warrior Actions at the end of each chapter Breathe is one of the actions. It is also Day 1 of the 31 Days Healthier Happier programme and consistently gets good feedback about how much better people feel just taking a few minutes each day to focus on their breath.

I have also done other extensive work over the last few years using NLP, coaching and hypnotherapy to deal with the bigger stresses. For some people that type of treatment is sufficient, for others they may need more focused and more direct treatment and coaching.

As I mentioned before some stress is good for you – it's the hormone that wakes you up in the morning, creates health benefits of exercise, lets you feel excitement, makes you aware of danger, sometimes a bit of pressure to meet a deadline is just what you need to stay focused – getting a report (or in my case a book) written on time, getting the kids out the door to school/activities on time...

We have created a world where we are accessible 24/7 and 365(6) days a year... With phones and technology we embrace it because it can make life easier and gets things done faster but on the other side of that we have created a monster for ourselves not being able to switch off, not respond to emails or messages when we are supposed to be on a day off or on family time and then we feel guilty about taking back control of our happiness if we try to switch off. And when we contact people there is a level of expectation that they should be instantly responding.

A popular trend seems to be emerging for people to wear their stress and exhaustion as a badge of honour/ status symbol to prove how hard working they are... 'I was up till 3 am working' 'I live on 4 hours sleep a night' 'you can rest when you are dead' or 'work hard, play hard', 'everyone needs me and I just can't ignore them' or 'I just don't have time'.

This mind-set and action is not good for your stress levels or health, the only thing it is going to do is be a contributing factor in ill health or premature death (yes, that drastic). It is almost seen as shameful if you are taking time out to do fun and relaxing stuff without your phone being glued to your hand... What we need to do is change that way of thinking, make work time focused on work and rest time focused on rest.

For us women if we are not doing it all (career, family, fun) and looking amazing (perfect hair, makeup, clothes, body) while doing it... well we should be ashamed of ourselves for letting it slip... Kiss. My. Ass. We are real, we are human, we are amazing but we are not Stepford Wives.

Who defines that image anyway? We can blame the media or celebrities or TV but once again we need to take responsibility for the pressure that we put on ourselves. Be confident about who you are, what you look like and wear your beauty with pride, makeup or no makeup, hair brushed or hair wild, a flat stomach or soft round the edges. Striving to look like a photo shopped image from the internet is one stress that we can all do without.

How often do you take some down time and feel guilty about it? Maybe all you are doing is sitting on the sofa having a tea or coffee and in your head all you can think about is the washings that need to be put on, the hoovering, and the emails, whatever is not allowing you to just sit in peace because it all feels like a priority. In the past I would get agitated if I sat down to chill... but now not as much as I used to. There are still times when I sit down and I remember the washing needs to be hung, dishwasher needs emptied or floors need mopped (the joys of living alone). You need to let go of this need to be superhuman and perfect all the time. It's exhausting and slowly killing us. So what if the house is a bit untidy for another 15 minutes?!

It can be really easy to blame external sources for

your stresses; our boss is demanding deadlines are met, your partner is wanting time with you, the kids need help with their homework, extended family and friends want some of your time, work, the government, the weather, the bus/train driver, the shopkeeper... It's anyone and everyone else's fault and they all want a piece of you.

With that in mind, the first thing we have to do is take responsibility for ourselves and our own actions.

It's your fault... (harsh but true, we need to take responsibility). That doesn't mean that you take everything on your shoulders and think of yourself as a failure. This is about you taking responsibility and control of your own happiness. Say 'yes' to more of the things that make you happy and life easier and 'no' to things that don't make you happy or drain your time and energy. And ask for help. It is easier to play the blame game, but the reality is we are trying to do too much and try to show up as perfect all the time. You are human, and that means you are not perfect and your environment is not perfect and life isn't perfect, so you need to let go of this particular stress and be a bit imperfect.

Breathe, yes I said be a bit imperfect, this comes from a former 'perfectionist'. I am not suggesting that you just stop giving a shit but take the pressure off a bit, give it your best effort each time and know that is all anyone should expect of you.

You are in control of you and your life and you can take yourself out of a situation or change your reaction to it at any time. First you need to breathe and assess the situation. My favourite question to ask myself and get my clients to ask themselves when they find themselves in a stressful situation is:

What is the best way I can deal with this situation right now?

It is up to you to say 'no' when it means you are putting yourself out by saying yes. It is up to you to switch off your phone/laptop, and not be available on demand. And it is up to you to detach yourself emotionally from a situation you have no control over (like when it is dealing with someone else's emotions or reactions).

If your boss keeps loading work on to you, it's probably because you are so freaking awesome and they trust you but it's also because you keep saying 'yes'. You need to let them know that yes you are an amazing human being and now that you are becoming a Warrior Woman you are not pretending to be superhuman anymore... You, your happiness and your health are way more important.

If the kids want to be part of every after school club and activity going, it is up to you to decide what and where you can reasonably get to or team up with other parents to share the responsibility of taking turns to take them. One of my friends has a strict rule that after

8pm it is her time and her kids have learned that they need to respect that or deal with the consequences of a really grumpy mum – there is some flexibility there when it is needed but it works really well for them as a family to have set those boundaries and respect.

There may be people in your life that are constantly demanding time and support from you and you don't seem to ever get any in return, have you been there as Miss Fix It? Looking for their problems, solving the problems, giving advice, holding their hands, loving them, caring for them, picking up after them – you get a real sense of being needed but when it starts to be taken for granted and you are getting stressed and emotionally drained, you need to learn to say no and find your own support...

The people around you are not mind readers, not your boss, your kids, your partner, friends or anyone else. You need to speak up ask for help yourself and you need to learn to stop fixing everything, they need to learn for themselves, and they will manage. As a Warrior Woman you are there to be a leader, to guide them to solving their own stuff, believe me, they will thank you for it later when they have been inspired in to becoming a Warrior Woman (or Warrior Man, they can be trained) for themselves.

The government... What can we say... They do their thing, we need to do ours. Maybe one of you Warrior

Women has aspirations to lead the country... What is it that is stopping you for going for it? Maybe we need to take a leaf out of the Icelandic women's book and start going on strike to see if they listen to us then.

The weather... As Billy Connelly famously said, 'There is no such thing as bad weather, only the wrong clothes'. For those of us in the UK, it rains (a lot). This is nothing new, some summers are good, and some are bad... There really is nothing you can do except buy really cool all weather gear and a pretty umbrella.

When it comes to dealing with other people, it is worth remembering that everyone has their own problems and their own shit to deal with. I don't want to burst your bubble but the truth is other people are so wrapped up in themselves and their own problems that you won't be their highest priority just like they shouldn't be yours. If people are rude, in a bad mood or give bad service, understand that they might have something else going on or that they haven't found the Warrior Woman Project to help them feel better (you can always pass on the book or link to the book for them to buy – shameless plug).

If you have ever done anything a bit mad and out of character or afterwards thought 'what the hell made me react like that / do that / say that?' it has likely been something else completely stressing you out, blocking your brain and clear thought processes. You know things like, sending a text/email in haste, throwing things out the window (my old neighbours used to do that a lot), throwing a drink over someone, saying something you don't mean, standing up and forgetting instantly what you were going to do, buying the wrong milk, impulse shopping, binge eating, generally making silly mistakes. I think it's fair to say that we have all at some point at least once reacted to something like that list, well that is stress taking control of you instead of you taking control of the situation.

Brilliant I can hear you say, but what can we do to start to take better control?

Exercise

There are many ways to combat stresses depending where your source comes from and everyone has different success with different things. Try each of these different techniques to see which ones are most effective and best suited for you. What is good for one is not necessarily good for another.

Breathe. The best thing about this exercise is you can do it absolutely anywhere and at any time.

* Think about how you breathe right now. Just notice it. Be aware. Are you just breathing in to the top part of your chest? (it's common to just breathe in to the top part of our chest when we are not thinking about it, are really busy or are stressed).

* Start to slow your breathing down. Try and fill your lungs, let your rib cage move out the way and your belly relax then slowly let that breath out as fully as you can.

* Do this for 3 full breaths. When you are breathing out as fully as you can, you are clearing out the stale air that sits at the bottom of the lungs.

* Start counting your breath, count how long it takes you to fully breathe in and how long it takes you to fully breathe out. Once you

have your number (most people are somewhere between 3 & 8) match your inhale
and exhale to be the same count, make is as
smooth as you can.

* It doesn't matter how long your breath is,
it's what feels comfortable for you. Through
practice it will naturally get longer but that
is not the aim of this exercise it is just to
follow the breath in counting and out counting.

Do this as often as you can, for about 5 minutes when
you wake up, when you are sitting in traffic, on your
commute to work, after a difficult phone call or meeting
(before if you know you are going in to a difficult call
or meeting), while you are on the toilet, waiting for the
kettle to boil, while you are reading...

That exercise is a form of meditation, taking your
mind away from everything else and just focusing on
your breath settles, calms and clears your mind allowing you to deal with everything else better. You may
even find that you get better ideas, do better work and
are more creative.

Adjust your physiology & posture (how you are
sitting or standing) will have a big impact on your mood
and stress. Think about how you sit or stand when you
are feeling down, low in confidence, and sad... Your
head is down, shoulders rounded, hunched forward.

It is really difficult to breathe properly in this position. How do you sit at your desk, in the car, huddled under your umbrella, or when you are on your phone???

Then think about how you sit or stand when you feel good, chest lifted, shoulders back and open, up straight – You need to do more of this right here, right now and make a habit of it.

* Sit or stand up straight
* Relax your shoulders away from your ears
* Tuck your chin slightly in so your ears are over your shoulders so your neck is nice and long.
* Draw your shoulders back so the shoulder blades are sitting comfortably on your rib cage, this should open your chest allowing you to breathe easier.
* Lift and narrow your waist without allowing the ribs to lift up, this should make you feel taller and narrower – this should just be a light engagement not a full contraction so you can't breathe smoothly.
* Hold your pelvis in a neutral position (hip bones and pubic bone are in alignment with each other – use the heel of your hands on your hip bones and middle fingers in towards your pubic bone to check the alignment)

* Whether you are seated or standing place your feet and knees hip width apart (roughly a fist distance between your knees) and try to have your weight evenly distributed between the right and left.

* Breathe, your body should feel comfortable and relaxed in this position with no tension or pressure being held anywhere other than your core to support your posture.

Reduce your use of technology. Everyone finds this challenging particularly at first if you are a reach for your phone every 2 mins kind of woman. Once you have done it a couple of times and notice how much better you feel you will want to make sure you are fitting in some time every single day.

* Have 1 day a week that you can go as technology free as possible, or even have set times of the day you do and don't use it (like meal times, family time, down time).

* Read books instead of social media

* Go for walks (fresh air is amazing for stress reduction)

* Go on a road trip

* Meet friends or family for coffee, lunch, dinner.

* Connecting with nature and/or animals and/or people in real life is an amazing stress reliever and fun (when you are with the right people).

* Take yourself out of your 24/7 contact world, set new rules for yourself to use technology less every day.

Don't re-live drama. When someone or something upsets you, acknowledge your feelings and then move on. If you keep thinking or talking about what happened you keep the emotions running, 'You won't believe what he/she just said/did to me... blah, blah, blah'. The more you re-live the worse the emotion feels because you keep topping it up and you stay in that negative state longer. Let the past be the past. This includes road rage, breathe through it.

When you feel a negative thought or emotion coming up, acknowledge what the emotion is and why you are experiencing it (sometimes we are allowed to be sad or angry, we just want to avoid wallowing in the pain) then if it is appropriate to move on from that emotion do something to distract yourself. An emotion only lasts a few seconds, it is our mind and imagination that keeps it going and reliving it.

Write a gratitude journal. Research has shown that people who write and practice gratitude are happier and less stressed. The more you focus on the good things in your life that you are thankful for, the less stressed and more positive your thoughts stay. Get yourself a really special journal to write in with a good pen – and write in it. I have had notebooks in the past that I deemed 'too pretty to write in' and I was scared to make a mistake in them so didn't use them. It's just paper, make mistakes, nothing bad will happen.

* Every day write 3 things in the morning you are grateful for
* At the end of the day another 3 things.
* If you have more than 3 keep writing don't hold back

Doing exercise in some form of physical activity produces good stress which boosts your metabolism, grows muscles, improves bone density, improves sleep, reduces blood pressure and improves general health but if overdone it will create bad stress which is detrimental to all the benefits it can create.

If you are mentally exhausted, exercise is a perfect way to clear your head and let you feel re-energised because the brain uses a different part for thinking than it does moving and when you are concentrating on your exercises you don't think about anything else (just like when you are focusing on breathing).

Exercise becomes a problem when you work out at too high an intensity for too long, or you go back for another session too soon without a proper recovery, or you exercise without enough sleep/food/hydration or too many stimulants. If you go in to a session feeling weak and lethargic you will be doing more harm than good. Gentle exercise like Yoga, Pilates or walking are best when you feel that way but also feel like you really need to do something. Always listen to your body and if you start a workout and feel worse, stop doing it.

If you are unsure ask for help, get booked in with a personal trainer that advocates a good quality diet and rest times, if they operate a 'beast mode' or 'go hard or go home' policy I would advise you to avoid them. Watch how the trainers are with their clients in the gym, speak with the clients and other gym members about their experiences, and meet to have a conversation with the trainer before you sign up, make sure you like them and you feel a good vibe from them. Look at their social media pages, are they all about their clients and their results or is it all pictures of them flexing in the gym? That will give you a good indication where their priorities lie.

Smile. This is an amazing stress reliever, even if you don't want to smile, do it anyway. It sends signals to your brain that something is making you happy and all the right happy chemicals start to release lifting your mood. If your face genuinely does not want the corners of your mouth to turn up, hold a pencil or pen across your teeth so that the ends of the pencil are forcing the edges of your mouth out wide (just like a smile). It works ☺ . Even increase the smile to laughter, it is even more effective.

Warrior Action

* Meditate
* Reduce your use of technology
* If you have a work phone, switch it off when you are not on duty
* Ask for help
* Eat good healthy food
* Practice gratitude
* Exercise or move regularly
* Don't feel guilty for doing things that are fun
* Smile / laugh
* Give yourself a break
* Breathe

CHAPTER 6
WARRIOR RULE #5 FIND THE BALANCE

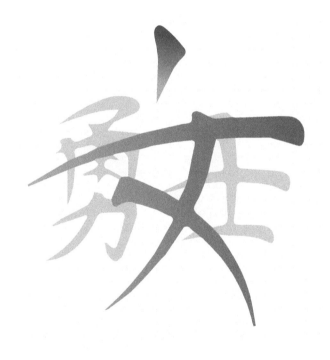

In life we have many different relationships and every single one has a different connection and purpose. Family, friends, lovers, work colleagues, bosses, people who serve us, people we serve, people we meet in passing and of course, ourselves.

There are a whole variety of them and we will connect to each of them in a different way and for different reasons.

Let me start talking to you about your energy (as in a vibe or flow rather than how energetic and enthusiastic you feel), this can be a lot to take in but please stay with me while I explain.

Every single one of us has a masculine and feminine energy – keep in mind that this has nothing to do with your physical appearance or sexual organs or sexual preference. It is to do with your energy and flow, how you think and feel and react to things particularly when you feel stressed or under 'threat'. Who you are at work can also be different to who you are at home as well as who you come in to contact with.

Masculine energy (alpha): driven, focused, analytical, decisive, leaders, deliver, fixer, linear, logical, has a need to complete or finish a task, competitive, want to sort things out to make people happy, stop at nothing – think Sarah Connor (Linda Hamilton) in Terminator 2 or Miranda Priestly (Meryl Streep) in Devil Wears Prada.

Feminine energy (beta): emotional, likes to talk and feel feelings, emotions, intuitive, go with the flow, don't like to make decisions, breezy, receivers, creative, multi-taskers, can have lots of unfinished tasks, passionate and like to work with others – think Holly Golightly (Audrey Hepburn) in Breakfast at Tiffany's or Mary Hatch (Donna Reed) in It's a Wonderful Life.

In an ideal world we would all have a balance of both and the ability to move between each to react and respond accordingly to your situation or other people we are in contact with. Many of us though, will most likely fall more strongly to one than the other to where feels most comfortable when we feel under pressure.

I default to masculine, I like to be in charge, I am independent, not good at letting people help me, I don't read instructions or ask for directions and I like things to be in order and analytical . God help anyone who tries to tell me who I am or what I want in life, if someone tries to alpha me (particularly if they don't know me), they generally get alpha Jen right back in their face. I will be majorly defensive and protective of myself and the situation (like keeping my business safe). This can be very different though if I am around a strong masculine energy that I fully trust and I will soften.

My mum, she is oh so feminine, she can be indecisive and likes other people to take charge and look after her, she also wants to offer solutions to all your problems and talk about feelings and she is so creative, she is a beautiful and talented painter.

Just because these are our default energies that doesn't mean that we don't have or can't access the opposing side. If I completely trust someone or if I am completely exhausted and just need someone to take over, I will allow them to take control of a situation. My best friend Grant is one of those masculine energies that get to be boss.

When we used to go on holiday as a family and even now when my mum and dad go away, my mum books the holiday, sorts all the packing and money, holds the tickets, passports, knows all the details of where and when to be, all my dad needs to do is turn up and carry the suitcase. She even took control and completely organised my wedding for me.

Our default is where we feel safe and comfy, and where we energise from. The opposing can sometimes feel like a challenge and a real effort and can be draining.

Your surroundings can also have an effect on the balance, if you think of a big city, towering buildings, straight lines, strong edges; the energy there is very masculine, it's busy and things get done in that city. People who have strong feminine energy might not feel comfortable there, even overwhelmed or being there might encourage the masculine side to come out a bit more.

On the other hand if you go out in to the country-side it can be very feminine energy, you are with nature where things are softer and flowing, things generally feel more laid back, calm and easy. Someone of a masculine energy may again feel uncomfortable there or they may allow themselves to freely release in to their feminine and kick back enjoying the more relaxed space.

In the ideal world we would move freely between each situation and be comfortable there. I found learning about this stuff helped me understand why I was the way I was in each environment and around different people and it has helped me feel more relaxed about moving between the energies.

So how do you know which you fall to?

When you are feeling stressed out or are out of your comfort zone have a look at your actions;

How do you react?

When do you feel most comfortable?

What's happening in your world when everything in it feels right?

For us ladies who are more masculine energy, you like to be the boss and in control, and independent and if you have the wrong understanding of being feminine (which for a long time I did) you can feel like you are weak and inadequate (especially asking for help) but this is not the case, vulnerability is a beautiful and courageous strength (so I have learned).

I remember seeing somewhere (probably social media) a quote:

'You must trust that the feminine side of yourself is not stupid, inadequate or weak.'

This really stopped me in my tracks as I had always identified that asking for help or admitting I couldn't do something was a sign of weakness. Being open and creative and allowing other people to make decisions is actually a really powerful energy to have AND it can also help release some of the stress that we put ourselves under.

For the feminine energy ladies, being confident and taking control of a situation and becoming a bit more decisive and competitive is not going to scare people away from you. In fact (wo)maning up from time to time is not a bad thing and it is great to boost your confidence as you learn your strengths. You have got your big girl pants, now put them on, pull them up and enjoy the power this energy flow gives you.

As a Warrior Woman you need to respect and live both sides of the energy which can be a small learning process for some and a massive learning curve for others. If something in the past has happened that has pushed you more strongly in to one of those energies then working on believing and trusting yourself is going to be a big part of the process of finding better balance.

So, how do you become a bit more balanced?

First thing would be going back to learning to love yourself more (we go in to this in detail in Chapter 8). When you love and trust yourself you discover strengths you maybe didn't realise or remember you had. You can soften and ask/accept help becoming vulnerable or stand up for yourself, showing the world you are a strong, confident, independent Warrior Woman with your big girl pants on.

There will be people who bring out the opposite in you to allow you that better balance, values will be aligned and it will work nicely. For the masculine warriors, there will be people in your life who are masculine energy and you trust and allow them to charge and do things for you... Let them take care of you. Or in the opposite; for the feminine warriors, there will be people who need you to 'man up' and take control of situations and do it... Show yourself and the world that you can be the boss and you will live the Warrior Woman ethos. Go back to your values and work with what is right for you in each situation.

Once you get your head round the different sides of the energies and understand who you are, who other people are and what roles the other people are in your life fill it lets you understand your relationships a bit better.

You will start to learn how to be with other people to bring the best out of them and bring the best to the situation to make it work.

If you have 2 feminine energies running a business, the creative ideas are going to be amazing, but one of you needs to take control and bring the masculine energy to the table to make sure that tasks get completed. Likewise if you have 2 masculine energies, there may be times one of you has to soften to the feminine to bring creativity in and allow things to flow.

If you are a mum at home there will be times that you need to be masculine to get the kids ready and wherever they need to be and other times that you allow your feminine energy to flow and let them be kids.

If you are in a relationship understanding each other's roles within the relationship can help that work and flow much better.

Masculine & Feminine Energy

Masculine		Feminine
driven		emotional
focused		intuitive
analytical		flowing
decisive leaders		indecisive
linear		breezy
logical		creative

Consider where you are on the scale, are you more one that the other or are you fairly balanced?

It can be easy to be balanced when things are going well, you will be more aware of a shift when you feel threatened or stressed and your fight or flight defence system or run and hide while other people sort this out kicks in. And that is okay, work with your strengths but be mindful of how it is impacting the situation. If you are locking heads with someone or a decision can't be made something needs to change to improve the situation. Because you are learning and understanding about this stuff, you are once again going to take responsibility and help make the situation as easy as possible.

Once you know where you sit, think about the relationships you have in your life.

Understanding the balance can really help improve your relationships and contact you have with everyone.

There are always going to be people who really motivate, inspire, make you feel amazing and you look forward to spending time with them, you leave feeling energized and excited about life. These will likely be the people that balance and work well with your energy whether they let you be the masculine or feminine and it will just fit and flow nicely.

At the opposite end of the scale there will be people you dread seeing, they can bring out the negative, insecure and exhausting feelings. These will be the people who challenge your energy. Maybe it is two masculine clashing heads or two feminine where neither will decide about anything or even one masculine and one feminine that can't find the right balance and wind each other up.

Then there will be the others somewhere in between, maybe sometimes balanced, sometimes completely out of balance. Maybe you can only deal with each other when you are both in a particular frame of mind…

I found understanding this really helped me understand others, work better with others and know when to let some things go to make certain relationships work better. There will always be people that you have to deal with that will challenge you and there sometimes is no getting round it when there is a clash. As I said before, you are now empowered with this knowledge and you can use it to a positive advantage (but not to manipulate in a deceptive way).

It would be easy for me to just tell you to spend lots of time with the positive impacting people and no time with the negative people. In the realistic world that isn't going to be the case and it's not necessarily a bad thing. You get to learn, you get stronger, you become more resilient, and you will improve your patience. The good news is though that what we have learned about ourselves through the last 5 chapters and what we now know about masculine and feminine energy balance we are now better equipped to deal with them. Upskill all the way.

Energy is one part of people and their make-up, another is our values which we have already looked at back in Chapter 2. If you find you have people who are draining, or forcing you across energy systems that don't work for you, you can look at the values that are being misaligned for you, and work out how you can make the situation better for both of you.

For example if someone is forcing their masculine energy and you feel disrespected when respect is a high value, matching their masculine energy and having a conversation about respect could be an effective way of dealing with the situation. If you matched that masculine energy with a feminine energy and started talking about your feelings there is a chance (depending on the person) that you will be met with resistance.

Regardless of whether or not there is conflict with others it is important to create boundaries within your relationships. It helps with conflict where sitting down and having a conversation with them to try and get them to see and understand what and why the situation isn't working for you. I always find honesty is the best policy. Some people are completely blind to the fact that there is even a problem. When there is no conflict in a relationship, having boundaries always allows you to have your own space and everyone knows where they stand.

Having this understanding can help you be more adaptable, build better relationships with others and also help you improve and manage the more challenging ones. Remember that you are only responsible for your own actions and reactions, not anyone else's.

NB. Please remember and use this understanding of energy for the greater good of all your relationships and NOT to manipulate or have power over others (I have seen this in action and it is ugly).

A Warrior Woman always lives by her values.

The most important relationship you need to have and work on is with yourself, this is the only one that you have total or any control over and the first step to doing that is understanding who you are and why you are the way you are.

When we think back over the previous chapters and you are living to your values, following your dreams and goals, letting go of the self-sabotage, dealing with your stress and then include this chapter of balance you can absolutely accept yourself, make friends with the part of yourself you don't like and actually learn (if you don't already) to love yourself.

When this is in place you will set standards of how you expect to be treated, people see how you treat yourself and match that respect. You are the leader of your own life setting the example to everyone and anyone around you learning from you (and if you ever get the honour to discover the number of people that you have an impact on, you will be blown away). You will be the teacher to others and there will be a mutual level of respect from them.

Warrior Action

* Understand your energy balance
* Align it with your values
* Be aware of the balance in relationships with others
* Take responsibility for your own energy
* Give yourself a break
* Breathe

CHAPTER 7
WARRIOR RULE #6
STOP CLEANING, START CREATING

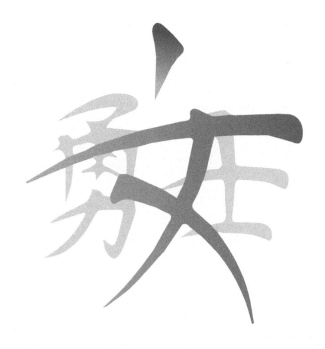

Jen Wilson

How many times do you find yourself putting things off, stalling, 'I will do it later', 'I will start tomorrow', 'I will start on Monday/next week/1ˢᵗ Jan' ignoring calendar reminders, re-prioritising because the other thing is just so much more important, waiting for someone or something else to do their bit or waiting for the right time?

I have news for you... Now brace yourself...

Things only happen when YOU take action. Yikes!

The good news is though you are not alone in the world of procrastinators; procrastination is something that we talk about a lot at workshops and courses. I also asked in the Warrior Woman Project Facebook group 'what do you do when everything feels like a priority?' Every single answer came back with some sort of procrastination or panic and run away response.

If procrastination was an Olympic sport I am pretty sure I would be in with a good chance of a gold medal. It is always the things that challenge us and push us out our comfort zone that we are happiest to avoid.

When I was at university my house must have been the cleanest house inside with the clearest windows on the block. It only took me to my final year studying, to work out that I would have heaps of spare time and a whole lot less stress if I stopped with the excuses and just got the work done.

When I was to do a video link for the Warrior Woman Project it took me about 4 months to actually do it, I had all the excuses, my roots needed done, my fringe was too long, I had the wrong top on, my skin wasn't looking great, I forgot, or the laptop was playing up... In the end... 37 seconds of video I did it and I put it online.

The main reason for the delay was I didn't want people to see me, which is stupid because they need to see me. I have an amazing course that helps women find balance in their life, be better versions of themselves and overcome their fears... there was one of mine right there. I faced the fear, and it turned out okay (that is one of those risks that I was talking about in chapter 4).

Once you get over yourself and just do what needs to be done, you actually feel pretty damn good and more confident... Proud even.

Procrastination is something that we have mastered over the years and it is also something that probably infuriates us the most.

When it comes to overcoming procrastinations, the questions I get asked the most are:

* How do I stop procrastinating?
* How do I stop my To Do list overwhelming me?
* How do I get motivated to just get stuff done?

Now, I am not about to pass you a get out of jail free card here, however, sometimes (just sometimes) we need to procrastinate to get the best result out of ourselves. You sometimes need to take a bit of time to get your head clear and make sure that what you are doing is the right thing for you at that time and not just jumping in without thinking about anything (4 months for a 37 second video was not an acceptable amount of time). Sometimes that delay can teach us more about who we are and make sure we are in the right place when we do take action. On the other side of that though, taking action and failing can also be the lesson that we need to take us to the right place.

So there is one of the challenges around procrastination; how do you know when to hold back and when to take the leap of faith?

Making decisions can be tough... I believe that our decisions are always the right ones, even when they don't turn out how we want them to. The job you didn't get, the boy who knocked you back, the dress that isn't available in your size, the holiday that you didn't go on – none of them were meant for you and better things will come when the time is right. That doesn't give you the get out of 'what's for you won't go by you', everything will go by you if you are sitting back and not taking any action waiting for 'the right moment'. In taking action you get to experience a whole lot more.

If you often find yourself thinking 'could've, should've, would've' then you are regretting the decisions you didn't make (although, by not making a decision you are still making the decision to not take action).

If you find yourself feeling overwhelmed by making a decision or taking action you are letting fear para- lysing you from progressing through life towards those dreams and goals that we have previously talked about.

So what do we do when we find ourselves most of the time faffing about, or delaying decisions, or avoiding responsibility? How do we get over these feelings of being overwhelmed or fearful?

Exercise:

Take a big deep breath, and stop thinking about whatever it is you are trying to achieve and focus just on your breath. As soon as you find your mind start to wander, bring it back to your breath. Spend a few moments here just breathing, allowing your mind to calm and settle.

Once you start to feel calmer and more settled from a distant view point start to make a list or look at your To Do list to establish what it is that needs to be done or decided.

* What part of the thing is it that you are really avoiding?
* How can you break that down a bit more to make it seem like less of a daunting task?
* Are there genuine pros and cons to the outcome?

Keeping in mind the best case scenario, make a list of all the positive outcomes that will come from completing the task or making the decision, have this list include both the emotional and material positives.

For example on my task of being creative daily the positive outcomes for me include: peace, calm, de-stress, vulnerability, business productivity, increased income and learning.

Then I would like you to think about what will your world look like when you have completed the task? Add that to your list, hopefully you are writing it down to make it more effective, clear and powerful but if it's a mental note then take time to think about that too.

Something that I haven't mentioned before is tapping in to your imagination. I would like you to imagine the future. Close your eyes and visualise the completed task, jump right to the end point where everything is done, don't think about the journey you may or may not take to get there, have the focus just on the final goal. Get a really clear picture of this in your mind, think about what you would see, what you would hear, what you would feel, really tap in to your senses here, maybe even what you would smell or taste might be relevant here too. The clearer the picture the more effective this exercise will be.

This task in itself may be considered a form of procrastination but it is productive procrastination that helps you get a clearer understanding of the 'what' and 'why's'.

Once you have that clear in your head, have a think about what needs to be done based on the importance of it. When you go to your list and start taking action, set yourself a short time frame, for the next 20 minutes that one task is all you are going to do. I have always found that once you get started it is easier to keep going, and before you know it you are ticking off that list and getting things done.

For some people their working environment is really important and they can't start working until their space or working area is clear, clean and tidy. If this is you, make sure that you create that space in advance, maybe the night before and make sure that you can't use that as an excuse in the morning. If the ritual of tidying puts you in to your headspace for work then make that part of your list and start earlier.

The more we can plan ahead, set our following day up the night before, looking at your list, knowing what it is that you need to do, then setting up your space so that you are limiting the potential excuses for the next day.

It is important to find a way or an environment that allows you to get the work done. When I started writing this book I needed to be away from my house and in a café where I didn't have good WiFi. The reviews and edits were slightly different, I found I didn't want to sit at my laptop so much so I bought a notepad and the 2nd edit started out handwritten and the final drafts were done at my kitchen table in short 2 hour bursts or train commutes to Birmingham for meetings.

There will be some things that you avoid because they bore you to tears or challenge you in unproductive ways, that is when you will very much benefit from learning the art of delegation...

I employed an assistant to make sure that all my emails and website are up to date, and all I need to do is write the content. She also does other amazing technical stuff that I don't really know what it is, I just ask for things and she makes it real for me. There is nothing I hate more than sitting at a computer waiting for websites to upload and moving between screens and what takes me about 3 hours to do, she does in around 20 minutes. There is also the additional benefit that she holds me accountable and when my content is not ready for her to upload she is chasing me up – at that point I need to stop procrastinating and get some work done.

Depending on what it is you need to be doing, getting a coach or mentor is extremely valuable. Not only do you have a sounding board to bounce ideas off of, but you also have someone holding you accountable. There is a coach or planner out there for just about every area of your life.

There will be times in life though when you just need to get away from everything to clear your head and chill out so that you can then make a better more productive start later. Allow yourself to have these times, give yourself room to breathe and clear your head. Some of the best ideas come through meditation, a long walk, a bath, going on holiday. Changes of scenery and surrounding yourself with different people will always help you see things from a different perspective.

On the other side of that though, as much as I want to give you permission to not beat yourself up all the time, there are times when you just need to pull your big girl pants on, put your phone away, switch off all distractions and do what needs to get done and deal with it.

This is your life, your happiness and your responsibility to make it the best that you can. Being pissed off with yourself and your excuses does not make you a happy Warrior Woman. Being pissed off with yourself can spur you in to action and stop making excuses, so if you need to, listen to her for a minute, get pissed at your situation, then start listening to your inner warrior and take the action you need to get where you need to go.

Procrastination at its worst is stalling, and holding back from whatever it is you want to achieve. Whether it is weight loss, finding romance, starting or pushing your business forward, moving to another country that you want for yourself.

All procrastination is, is you being controlling and wanting or needing everything to be perfect (this is said from a former control freak perfectionist who is working hard to changing her ways). Taking that first step and letting go of control can be scary, change can be scary; it can be outright terrifying, especially when we don't know what the outcome of the change will be. A new job, a career change, a new relationship, a new country to live in...

What we need to remember is that change is also the most amazing thing ever... Yes it can be scary but... a new job, a career change, a new relationship, a new country to live in... these can all fulfil your dreams and goals, create new exciting opportunities, show you a whole new world of experience that you would never get if you continued to avoid change.

No one wants to or deserves to live an unhappy or unfulfilled life. If you are genuinely unhappy in your life then you need to be brave and make the decisions you need to make to be happy again. Making the decision to end my marriage wasn't easy, that whole process took me to many unhappy places before I was truly happy again, most of that unhappiness was through my procrastination in dealing with my emotions. Ultimately if we had stayed together we would have both been unhappy staying in a marriage just to keep the other person happy. Maybe your decisions are bigger than that, maybe they are not, whatever they are at the core of it is you and your happiness.

When you think about the universe and planets in their entirety, in the grand scheme of things we are not on this planet for that long, and we are pretty tiny, so really we want to make what we have as happy, fun, interesting, and fulfilling as we can. Yes, that can be easier said than done... But you must be looking for something to be here and reading this book.

We need to live a life of fear of regret rather than fear of failure.

When you think about 'the end' (yeah, your last few breaths), no one gets to their death bed and says 'I really regret taking all those chances in life'. We never regret the chances we have taken, the only thing we do regret is the chances we didn't take (the boy you didn't speak to, the job you didn't apply for...).

When we have these fears the wrong way round we procrastinate more and regret more... Missed conversations, opportunities, connections... 'If only I had just spoken to / said that / had a go...' When you give it a go, at least you know the outcome instead of assuming the outcome.

So how do we get past this procrastination and fear of change to start embracing it?

Exercise

Similarly to the previous exercise, start with a few big deep breaths in and out, keeping your focus as much as you can on your breath until you feel a sense of calmness.

Then, I want you to have a look at where you are in your world right now.

> What is it specifically about your world is it that you don't like?

So often we take the focus just on to the dream and don't think about the place that we are at right now, sometimes it's not actually that far from where you want to be or it is so polar opposite it propels you into action. Get right down to the tiny details. This is not to put you in to a bad mood, but to get you to realise what it is exactly that you don't like.

Is it something you have control over?

If it is something that is within your control, what can be done to change it?

Often when you start to break it down to the specifics it can be one small aspect that seem to be fixated on and it brings you down. Change what you can.

If you are not happy with your job, lifestyle, hairstyle, makeup, fashion – change it, there are so many people out there that have created businesses out of helping people make change. Find someone that in their videos or in their blog posts speaks your language, gets what your problem is, feels like they are already inside your head looking at the world through your eyes. If you feel sluggish and distracted and could do with a boost to your energy levels – change what you are eating, make sure there are lots of healthy choices in there, make sure you are drinking enough fluids, and seek out professional advice if you need it.

I know several people who read and listen to every personal development and self-help books, videos, podcasts, courses etc. that is around. They are gatherers of information, the thing is, they never actually do anything with all the information that they are gathering. You can read and listen to and agree with them all, but if you don't take action and change something, nothing is going to change.

Be the one that makes the change and inspires other people.

Warrior Action

* Get over yourself, don't let your ego hold you back
* Understand that everyone has these same issues
* Takes some time to think about what it is you actually want (go back to your goals from chapter 3)
* Make a list, plan ahead and schedule in your time
* Take action
* Find an accountability buddy
* Find a coach or mentor that will help you
* Reward yourself for completing tasks
* Give yourself a break
* Breathe

CHAPTER 8
WARRIOR RULE #7:
SELF-LOVE, BELIEVE IN YOURSELF

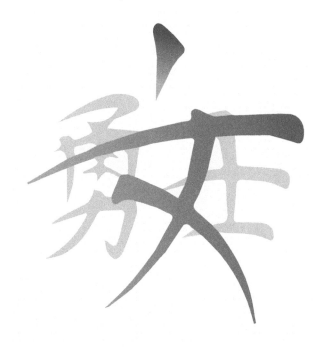

Although I believe that self-love is different from self-belief, I do think that they go hand in hand and one is as important as the other which is why I have put them both together in one chapter. You could have elements of one without the other but they are much more powerful together.

When I think about self-love, I believe it is about looking after yourself, respecting yourself, putting yourself first, and filling your cup (that cup of water that I talked about in chapter 1). Self-belief knows that you can do it, it's the confidence behind the actions.

I know someone (several women actually) that look after themselves in terms of clothes, hair and make-up but struggle with their weigh. They are beautiful and always well-presented but are really not happy with their weight, social life and / or relationship status. They have enough self-love to present themselves to the world in a particular way, and they have enough self-belief to have awesome jobs, but not enough self-love or self-belief to take action to be happy in the other areas of their life.

You may be really fortunate to have people in your world who do believe in you and encourage you, that's great, start listening to them because not everyone has that kind of support around. The name itself 'self-belief' means that you need to be validated by the self rather than external sources. At first as you start to go through this process listening to the people who are telling you that you are good enough is important to help start to build your confidence. On the other side of that you need to not listen to the people who are telling you that you are not good enough. Maybe something isn't for you, but the best way to know for sure is to go after it and fail.

I have been very fortunate that my parents have always been supportive and encouraging; they stayed far enough back to let me make lots of mistakes and learn for myself but also were there when I needed them. At school I was always under the radar, middle of the road, and generally disengaged. 12 years I dawdled through with only a couple of teachers for a few sporadic classes that actually had me engaged and interested in their classes. I left high school not sure who I was, no idea what I wanted to do and thinking I wasn't good at anything.

Even now as a fully grown adult, loving what I do, I have questioned my abilities and even when others have told me I was good, it still needed me to validate myself to have self-belief. I look to my mentors and coaches for feedback any time I can. It is human nature to want someone to pat you on the head and tell you that you are doing a good job. It means even more when you get it without looking for it.

Just before completing this book I was notified of being nominated for 2 different awards, one of them I shortlisted as Mentor of the Year with Business Women Scotland and the other Best Pilates Instructor Glasgow with MoveGB, at the time of going to print I know I didn't win the Mentor of the Year but I don't know the outcome of the Pilates instructor one but am delighted to be recognised for my work.

I am a big believer in constructive feedback, it's how we learn, it's how we grow, it's how we gain confidence and self-belief and allows us to be better next time. Over the last couple of years I have become more confident, and I am realising that I do know what I am talking about. I can't tell you with 100% certainty whether the self-belief encouraged the self-love or the other way round, but what I can tell you is that over time, having worked through the content I have shared with you in the previous chapters, both have become stronger.

One particular fear I always had around self-belief was about coming across as being arrogant. Who am I to think I am great at what I do? The difference between arrogance and confidence is arrogance is fuelled by insecurity and there is an over compensation to try and prove you know what you are about. Once I understood this I was less concerned about sharing my knowledge and skills. You know what you know, share it and teach it with empathy.

When you are prepared to put the work in, learn the skills you need whether personal or professional, seek out the right people to ask for help, and take on board the constructive feedback to help you grow and develop and also acknowledge your successes so far, you have every right to have confidence and self-belief. If you are always looking for perfection to validate self-belief you are always going to be disappointed.

I remember reading a post on Instagram that said:

Good news.

You are perfect.

Everyone is.

Perfectly imperfect.

Embracing and accepting imperfections are all part of the process of believing in and loving yourself. I mentioned earlier in the book, vulnerability is one of your greatest strengths. If you believe and love yourself enough to put something out there and accept that if it doesn't work out then you can adapt and change to improve the next time you are embracing imperfection and not being arrogant. That doesn't meant that you don't need to put in any effort, everything you do should always be the best you can give in that moment.

When we are trying to be perfect all the time it creates an environment that is really stressful and exhausting, as a recovering perfectionist I can contest to that. You just never feel like you are good enough or that you will ever be good enough, you set the bar high (which is a good thing to have high standards and expectations of yourself) but as soon as you get close you put it up another 2 steps. By doing this you are never allowing yourself to feel and enjoy the success of your achievements so far because you are always just focused on the next step. Stop for a moment and look back at how far you have come, life moves so quickly that we need to take time to appreciate our journey.

We all have things that we see in ourselves that we don't like (think back to the exercise from chapter 4), but if someone else was to look at you, they don't see what you see and it's likely not only the negative things you see – some people find crooked teeth, chubby cheeks, that you turn red when you are asked about something you don't know or that a rumpy dump ass endearing.

You are going to embrace your imperfections and make them your own, most other people are too busy worrying about their own imperfections to worry about yours*. I have news for you; you are only the most important person in the room to yourself, just like they are to them. Make friends with yourself, remember; how would you speak to your best friend? Speak to yourself with that same love and compassion.

* A short note on people being judgemental, most often when you find yourself judging someone else (or when you hear someone else being judgemental) have a think about the motivation behind it. Is it because you have gone in search of some validation about an insecurity that allows you to think or feel 'at least I am not as bad as them'? More often than not it is in there somewhere, that need to make yourself feel a bit better. Notice when you do it yourself and call yourself out on it. It's an ugly habit to get in to and certainly not a Warrior Woman ethos.

How free would you feel if you weren't judging yourself and thinking negatively about yourself all the time? How much love would you be showing yourself if you were to start to put yourself first (even just some of the time to start with)?

Imagine getting up in the morning and looking in the mirror and thinking 'yip, you have got this, you are amazing' rather than 'hair is a riot' or 'my skin looks awful'. For many of us this might seem out of reach and maybe starting with 'you are enough' is where you need to be just now (I know women who have written that across their mirrors in lipstick, how you want it to work for you is up to you, post-it notes are equally effective and less messy).

Let's have a look at how you look after yourself.

What is the first thing you do when you get up?

Many of us reach straight for the mobile phone; do you check emails / social media?

Make breakfast for someone else?

Look in the mirror and tell yourself how horrendous you look?

Start work?

Get other people up and ready?

Rush about?

When you wake up do you feel like you switch on for everyone else whether it's your partner, family, your customers or boss/colleagues?

Learning some self-love will let you be the first person you look after. Think how nice it will be to take some time to care for you first.

Exercise

In the morning after you wake up and you have meditated (remember the breathing and keeping focus on your breathing, aiming for around 5 minutes or more if you can every day).

I have already suggested you do this in previous chapters and I am hoping that the more I repeat it the more likely it is that you will take me seriously on this one, have it scheduled in as a daily ritual, even if you are just being completely mindful brushing your teeth. Set your alarm a little bit earlier if you need to and just take the time for you.

Then, sit quietly with your breakfast, even better if you can have it outdoors. If this feels like it would be impossible to do that on work days, make a starting point of doing it on your days off.

While you are sitting quietly I want you to think about your achievements, remind yourself of the successes you have in your life. Take time to read or listen to something that makes you feel good or inspired and calm (audiobooks and podcasts are amazing to have on an mp3 device hooked up to a speaker in the kitchen).

Once you do this once and appreciate how good it feels you will definitely make the time to do it as often as you can, I am now timing it in to my work days, a shorter time, but time all the same. Maybe you do this already when you go away on holiday, try to bring that feeling in to your real everyday life.

Now that we are bringing some peace and time in to your life, we want to look at building more confidence to go with the calm, loving you.

Think about the things you are least confident about right now, those things that you shy away from doing or shift from one days To Do list to the next hoping that they will just action themselves or they have been on there so long that you can bin that idea all together.

Maybe it is going on a date, maybe it is applying for a new job, starting your own business, getting your driving licence...

The best way to build confidence with anything is to become competent at something.

Look back at your life so far, how many things have you achieved, what skills have you built?

Even walking or reading would have started out as something you were incompetent at, over time building skills, practicing, learning from mistakes you would have become competent and gained confidence. In your job, you would have started out not knowing what you were doing, through training, learning, taking action, you have built competence and confidence. You are not born with the skills you have now.

Exercise

Having a think about your dream life either on the page, in a notebook or in your head answer:

How would I like each day to unfold?

What would I like to be focusing my energy and attention on, if I had any choice available to me?

What makes me feel happy?

What gets me jumping out of bed looking forward to the day?

What makes me feel balanced and settled?

What state of mind would I like to be in while I work?

What other aspects of my life do I wish to be paying more attention to?

If I was to make one change this week what would it be?

What skills or experience do I have from the past that I can use to help me move forward today?

What new skill do I need to learn to be able to gain more competence?

Once you have the answers to these questions it should give a clearer understanding of what you need to help you map out a plan to being someone competent and confident to have more self-belief. Maybe you already are and have just been too scared to admit it to yourself or maybe there are a couple of small changes you want to make...

Competence + Confidence = Self-Belief

Self-Belief + Understanding + respect = Self-Love

Warrior Action

* Let go of being perfect
* Know that you are enough
* Work on your competence to be confident
* Know that confidence and arrogance are not the same thing
* Let go of judgement of yourself and others
* Make friends with yourself
* Give yourself a break
* Breathe

CHAPTER 9

WARRIOR RULE #8:
IF YOU REALLY WANT THE CAKE, HAVE IT

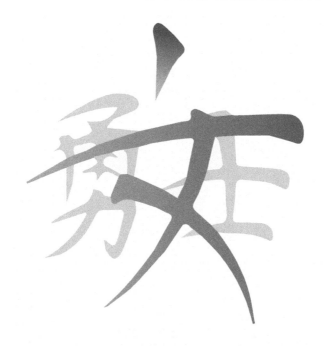

Talking about diets and eating is something I have recently added focus on within the Warrior Woman Project after noticing how often it came up in workshops and in coaching sessions. For many of the warriors, health or weight loss is one of their goals and more often than they realised is an area of their life that they self-sabotage in (you are not alone here, even I find myself doing this from time to time).

I also know through experience of working with many women over the years that food issues in some shape or form can come up even if they don't have a weight issue. Just about every woman I have ever spoken to knows exactly what I am talking about when I mention emotional eating.

Just in case you don't recognise that term, emotional eating is what we do when we are: stressed, sad, happy, angry, avoiding emotion, pissed off, hurt, rejected, anxious, depressed, bored etc...

Pretty much it is any time that you eat when you are not actually physically hungry. What you are doing is distracting yourself from a situation with food. This usually involves indulgent in foods that are not healthy, in large volumes, eaten unconsciously (without thinking and automatically) e.g. when you are watching TV eating a bag of crisps, you suddenly realise they are all gone and you don't remember eating any of them. It often can involve entire packets of biscuits, cakes, tubs of ice-cream, family bags of crisps and bottles of wine with a 'I don't care anymore, the world can kiss my fat ass' attitude.

Now, where this stems from is not exactly our fault or our parents fault, but it kind of is our parents fault when they (completely innocently) conditioned us to see food as comfort when we were small.

We were given sweets if we were good as a way of rewarding us, we got them when we were crying to keep us quiet or comfort us, or it was used as a bargaining tool to create desired behaviours. And then there was your grandparents and extended family filling you with cakes, biscuits, sweets because you were at your grans or aunties.

Apologies to the parents who have never used food as a reward, comfort or bargaining tool, but it does happen widely.

And I can't forget to mention the marketing companies who constantly show us images of women so happy and relaxed while eating bars of chocolate, girls having the best fun while drinking diet fizzy juice, how cool you are for drinking certain liqueurs, it's all sexy, cool, seductive and happy...

These emotional triggers have us believing, 'I have been good all week so I deserve....' 'I am sad so I will bloody well eat what I want' or one that was recently brought to my attention by a client 'I can afford to have this now; we didn't have the money when I was young', 'the woman in the ad is so beautiful when she is eating/drinking whatever'.

With all this in mind, I think it is appropriate to discuss it in this book.

For those of you who do have food or weight issues (that is even if you would just like your tummy to be a little bit flatter or your ass a little bit more toned).

How many diets have you tried?

You might not even want to start thinking about this, but how much money have you spent over the years on shakes, pills, tea, books, DVD's and you don't seem to be any closer to your goals? Maybe you are even further away from them?!

If you go in to a book shop or type diet book in to amazon there are thousands of books all promising you the perfect figure, guaranteed results and super-fast changes that may or may not be biologically impossible for you to achieve.

The supplement industry is the same. Tubs of all sorts of concoctions promising you to slim down, burn fat faster or bulk up.

The thing to remember is, if any of them actually worked then there would not be so many options on the shelves and not increasing numbers of people with health issues related to weight gain.

I read an article in a magazine once from an economist who reported that entire industries would collapse if every woman in USA and Canada stopped buying beauty and diet products for a week. These industries and their marketing teams pray on our insecurities and emotions to get us consuming optimistically.

My advice to every single person:

* **Stop 'dieting'** or following the latest fad or taking the latest miracle pill – removing food groups from your diet doesn't work, you need protein, fat and carbs from real food. Neither does replacing food with shakes. You might get a short term result, but seriously damage your health long term. Try to not think of foods as 'good' and 'bad', food is food and you want to eat it to nourish your body, mind and soul.

* **Eat mindfully.** Taking time to sit down and eat a meal instead of throwing food down our necks on the run or eating in the car on route to somewhere or watching TV while we eat. When we are distracted we don't register what we are actually eating, we often don't chew our food enough, meaning that your stomach isn't ready to digest the food and it hasn't been broken down enough before hitting out stomach. The problems there cause indigestion, heart burn and to a point can damage our body. When food that isn't broken down enough passes through, the nutrients can't be absorbed and our body can't do the job that it needs to. Turn off the TV, put away your laptop and phone. If you need background

noise (I am not a fan of hearing people chew) then put some slow paced music on in the background. Sit at the table if you have one. Use your knife and fork, but put them down between mouthfuls, don't load up your fork ready to go in as soon as you swallow. Chew your food, at least 20 times, get the saliva doing its work, make the task in your tummy easier and hopefully reduce indigestion or heartburn. Enjoy your meal, every mouthful.

* **Learn about food** and what works for you, this is mostly going to take time and be trial and error (don't learn from women's magazines, every month they change their mind, I have even seen contradicting advice within the one article). It's a minefield of information. Stick with lots of veggies, some fruit, good carbs in the form of oats, rice, veg, lean protein in the form of good quality meat, fish, eggs, tofu, beans & pulses, and fats from coconut oils, butter (not margarine), olive oils, avocados, oily fish, nuts, seeds, nut butters and oils. The more natural you can eat the better.

* **Think of it as creating a lifestyle** and be realistic about the changes, sort one thing at a time, integrate it with your life. An all-

out overhaul is too much for most people and will create a backlash when it gets too much, then you feel like a failure. Small manageable changes. If you have been eating coco pops for breakfast, then maybe your first change is to rice crispies or corn flakes if oats or eggs really don't cut it for you.

* **Create a mind-set with your goals and health** as your aim for success. Think about being healthy first. Eat food that makes you feel good inside and out. Food should nourish your heart and soul. If you eat something and instantly feel guilty... Why are you eating it? If you eat something that makes you bloat... Why are you eating it? If you eat something that makes your skin break out... Why are you eating it? You can see where I am going with this. Think about how you feel both mentally and physically. If you eat cake and you loved every mouthful and you felt good after eating it, then there really is no need to never eat cake.

* **Be around people** that will help educate you and support you and your goals. Those friends that take the piss or tell you that you need to let your hair down are only doing it because they don't have the same goals as

you or you make them feel guilty because they know they should be taking better care of themselves. You either need to have great support around you or be really strong minded to stick to it when the people closest to you are not on board.

* **Find activities and exercise** that you enjoy as a priority and mix it up from time to time. If you are not achieving your goals then maybe you need to change your approach – get help if you need it. Going to the gym and doing fitness classes is not for everyone. Try different things to see what you enjoy. There are loads of adult netball teams, walking, running, cycling groups around and many of them are free to join. Check out meetup.com for local groups in your area.

* **Understand why** there are things you don't want to have in your diet. Too much sugar can cause excess belly fat, can make you moody and breaks your skin out. Too much alcohol slows down the digestive system making you hold more fat and you usually eat a weeks' worth of junk food in the morning to get over the hangover. Processed food has a whole host of things added to it to make it taste good and be cheap to make, when things are far removed from their

natural state, your body struggles to use them and they have little to no nutrients to nourish your body and soul.

* **Keep well hydrated**; water, herbal tea, green tea, fresh made veg juices. It is recommended you drink around 2 litres of fluid a day, if you are always inside with heating or air conditioning these will dry you out more so you need more fluid, likewise if you are active for most of the day. Regular small sips of fluid all day is much better than glugging gallons in one go and then needing to pee it all out 20 mins later. Top tip, have water room temperature and if you do find you are peeing a lot a tiny pinch of sea salt in the water (not enough to taste) will help keep it in your body to be absorbed. If for medical reasons you are on a low sodium diet, this would not be recommended.

* **Get good sleep**. If you struggle to get to sleep at night get in to a routine. Turn off the laptop / TV at least 2 hours before bed (the light from the screen messes with the release of melatonin (sleep hormone) and keeps you awake longer. Chill out, have a bath, read, meditate, focus on your breathing making it slow and steady, make a bed time drink (I love Clipper Snore & Peace tea

or my healthy(ish) hot chocolate) you can get that and a collection of my favourite recipes here www.warriorwomanproject.com/recipes

* **Reduce your stress levels** – Go back to the chapter on stress, what else can you do to remove stress from your life? When you are stressed your digestive system doesn't work properly. I have found spending a minute before eating to focus on my breathing, taking long slow breaths for 6-10 repetitions calms me and has helped with the digestive process.

* **Make a treat a treat** – thinking back to the start of this chapter when I was talking about emotional eating, and eating as a reward. Things that should be considered 'treats' have become every day foods in our lives. Chocolate biscuits, cakes, crisps, take away food are all just there now as a convenience rather than a treat, we don't look forward to them. Resetting your connection with these types of food will allow you to have them as an occasional treat and you won't feel guilty having them. What is better: hiding behind the fridge door while you inhale half a cake feeling guilty, hoping

you don't get caught or sitting in a café with friends enjoying the chat and a bit of cake?

* Once we start to improve our relationship with food, we start to feel and look better. Always question your actions, is this for comfort or pleasure and health? Our skin is clearer, we have loads of energy, we sleep better, and as a bonus we look better. When the focus comes away from weight loss and what we look like to how we feel inside, our mood, our energy the stress of being the 'right' shape goes away.

We will never look like the girls in magazines (they don't even look like that thanks to Photoshop) and really if you knew the effort, stress, unhappiness they go through to look like that you would realise that to be really lean with your 6 pack showing is not a healthy way to be. Athletes look the way they do because their job is to be the best at whatever sport they compete in, that is their full time job. We can only look like us, we are all different shapes and sizes and a lot of that we have no control over.

What we do have is responsibility and control over is how we treat our bodies. We are fully responsible for what we eat and how much we move, accepting that responsibility and control can be the tough part. When you are on board with the rest of this book this will all seem so much easier.

Exercise

Now that we are starting to understand how food can be a benefit to us it will be really useful for you to start to track not just what you are eating but also how your food makes you feel. Start with a 3 day tracker including 2 working days and 1 non-working day. You can download your Food and Mood diary from www.warriorwomanproject.com/resources .

Remember to track food, drinks and portion size. How you identify portion size is completely up to you, it can be by weight if you have that information to hand or handful sizes. Whatever works better for you.

With your moods you are looking for energy levels increase, decrease, bloating, irritability, increase in happiness, decrease in happiness, cravings, sleep quality, how you feel when you wake up.

The more detail you take down the clearer your picture will be. If 3 days doesn't seem to be giving you a good enough picture, continue for 7 days, but don't get obsessed with it. Use it as an occasional tool to keep you focused, aware and on track.

So what do we do with that information? Depending on your goal and what you notice from your diary you can start to fine tune your lifestyle to make your food work for you. If you are noticing slumps in the day what have you eaten previously? If there is bloating or irritability, try removing certain foods and continue to monitor.

For further nutrition coaching I have a programme specifically designed to increase your knowledge and help you work towards making your eating work for you. Details are over at

www.warriorwomanproject.com/nutritionprogramme

Warrior Action

* Stop dieting
* Eat mindfully
* Learn about food and how it makes you feel
* Think of it as creating a lifestyle and be realistic
* Create a mind-set with your goals and health as your aim
* Be around supportive people
* Find activities / exercise that you enjoy
* Understand the why's of food you are eliminating
* Keep well hydrated
* Get good sleep
* Reduce your stress levels
* Make a treat a treat
* Give yourself a break
* Breathe

CHAPTER 10
WARRIOR RULE #9 LET GO

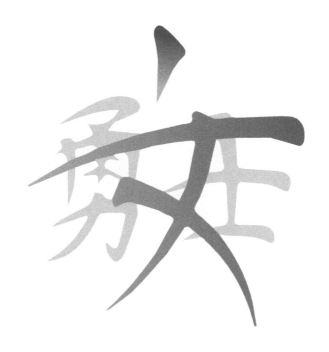

'It's your life, these are your goals. You control your happiness. Work hard, be honest with yourself, be kind to yourself and love yourself'

Jen Wilson Creator and Founder of Warrior Woman Project (yes, me).

When I was thinking about the Warrior Woman Project and discussing the idea with one of my mentors, they asked me some questions that really made me think about the programme and my vision; what would a Warrior Woman look like? What would their values be? What makes someone a Warrior Woman?

These are the values that I see in every Warrior Woman and maybe you have these on your list from Chapter 2 or maybe they weren't ones that particularly jumped out at you. Perhaps you haven't realised that you have these values or maybe you have not quite tapped in to them just yet (remember there is no hard and fast rule around these):

* Ability to let go
* Courage
* Determination

* Strength
* Freedom
* Warrior
* Love

It really and truly doesn't matter if your values list looks completely different to this list. Maybe some of these values you feel you still need to work on, maybe from working through this book you have realised that these are actually some of your values.

Let me explain to you Warrior Woman, how I see these fit in you as a Warrior Woman.

When you make the decision to let go whether it is of fear, anger, or control, then you tap in to our courage, you feel a sense of freedom and will feel happier. Think about the times you have held on to negative emotions, I am pretty sure that they won't have made you feel free or happy. If anything you will have felt more fearful, angrier or out of control. I was once told by a wise woman (my senior lecturer at college MaryAnn) 'control the controllable and let go of the rest'. You are the only controllable.

You can't be courageous unless you are taking some risks and in letting go there will always be some element of risk (or certainly a feeling of risk).

Have you ever considered though that the thought of changing a situation is worse than the experience and outcome itself?

If you are in a job you hate and you want to start your own business, the thought of not having the job security is scary but when you actually take the step and end up doing something you absolutely love doing you will find a happiness that can't be bought with cash. I tell you that from experience.

Maybe you can think about a time in the past when you changed job and really couldn't have been happier with that change. You left the security of a job you knew and the people you were familiar with to something where you were starting from scratch again learning a new system, possibly in a new location, and with a new team of workmates. Your new job and environment was amazing.

Sometimes a change is as good as a rest.

If you have been single for years and are very happy being single but you would quite like to be in a relationship the thought of finding that relationship is scary. Then you hear about other's dating disaster experiences which totally gives you the feeling of dread and despair that puts you right off even trying. The comfort of being single can be just too appealing. (This could be the same in the opposite; maybe being 'comfortable' but not happy in a relationship that isn't really what you want is easier than facing a life of being single).

Being open to the idea and accepting a relationship when it comes along for what it is, knowing that you were happy being on your own but this person adds a bit of happiness right now and if it doesn't work out that is still okay (remember you were fine before) can give you a whole lot of joy and open you up to something you weren't expecting.

Again, I speak from experience here. I was very comfortable being on my own, then one day this man appeared in my life through a chance meeting in Tesco. Cutting a long story short, a friend getting involved to move things in the right direction and somehow he just fitted and it all feels amazing. I know that it may or may not last, either way I have let go of trying to control anything, I am taking each day exactly as it comes and enjoying it for what it is.

The thing to remember when it comes to bringing someone else in to your life, whether it is a romantic interest or a new friend or a business partner, you need to be happy with who you are and what you want in your life so you can be independent in a co-dependent relationship. If you are trying to fill a void or are looking for someone else to make you happy, complete you, or fix you, then you are in the fast lane to having the wrong people around you. That's not to say that people can't be there for you and support and help you, but your motives for them being there need to be sincere to your needs and match your values.

It is the same thought process if you are in an unhappy relationship. Why are you unhappy? What is not happening for it to be happy? Maybe just going through the exercises in this book will be enough for you to realise who you are and what you want and that can change the dynamics of that relationship (this again can be friendships or family not just romantic). Sometimes the dynamics change for the better and you create something that works better and sometimes you need to walk away because it is the best thing all round for both parties (like my divorce and other connections I cut ties with over the years).

This courage gives you determination to keep going, to be strong and move towards our dreams and happiness. When you take the time to be clear on who you are and what you want it can make life so much easier to navigate through.

You can stand up and say 'Yes' to the things you want and 'No' to the things you don't want. You have confidence in yourself to have the strength in this powerful knowledge of you.

That gives you freedom and happiness. You know that through your hard work and honesty throughout the exercises in this book that you have sorted your shit out (and don't stress if you read that last statement and are thinking 'well not quite yet', you are a work in progress. I am a work in progress. We are not done until we are done (last breath done).

So what does it mean to have freedom? For everyone it can look slightly different but what I want to share with you is this.

In freedom you can look at yourself in the mirror and know that you are enough, that you are more than enough, you are awesome. Even if you don't quite feel it yet, you are well on your way. You can look yourself in the eye and see the Warrior Woman looking back at you with love. That love is who you are completely and what you have become.

You are a Warrior Woman.

Believe it will happen, then, work your ass off making it happen.

Exercise

I have created a video and audio download for you to help you let go. This is a lovely and very effective meditation to help you let go of stresses and tensions that you might be holding on to. To download this final exercise head over to

www.warriorwomanproject.com/resources

Warrior Action

- * Let go (use the download)
- * Use your courage
- * Allow yourself freedom
- * Love yourself
- * Give yourself a break
- * Breathe

CHAPTER 11
CONCLUSION AND MOVING FORWARD

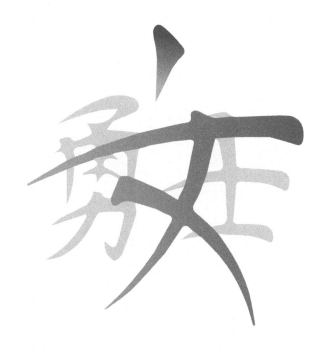

What happens now?

Firstly CONGRATULATIONS for getting through the book, all the way to the very end! Not everyone will have made it to this point, so be proud of yourself for this completion. It shows real determination and strength of character to push through. I know that some of the exercises will have challenged you (they challenge me too, but that's the point).

I personally would like to thank you for making it all the way through and genuinely hope that you got as much out of the process as I have done over the last few years. Rebuilding my life and finding confidence in myself and my abilities has been a journey and a half, and it's not over yet. It's not always easy and there will be slip ups, diversions, road bumps, challenges and life getting in the way from time to time. The more you stay focused on you and what you want, the more resilient and confident you will become.

If you are thinking that you are getting somewhere but you just need to get over a bump and don't think you can do it on your own then head over to

www.warriorwomanproject.com/sortyourshit

for details and a very special coaching offer just for those of you who made it this far. You can of course head back and repeat any of the chapters that you feel would benefit you. Working directly with me to coach you through will get you faster results than trying to go it alone so check out that special offer.

Remember that you are allowed to try as many things as you like in life. Don't think of anything as a failure; instead think of it as confirmation of something that wasn't right for you. I have 'failed' at so many things (school, businesses, a marriage, friendships, relationships...). There are so many things that I could probably write a whole book just on discovering what wasn't for me.

You will get to where you want to be because I know you want to (you read this book for a reason and got this far) and when you have worked out what it is you want, the planning and action phase just put all the pieces in place ready for you to take action.

Then you take the action, I have faith in you Warrior Woman...

With love,

Jen x

PS. If you have enjoyed this book can you please leave me a review over on Amazon and recommend it to your friends, family, work colleagues, or anyone that you think would benefit from the book, even buy them all it as birthday and Christmas gifts.

References

Colonel Chris Hadfield – The Sky is not the Limit (talk)

Brené Brown – The Power of Vulnerability (book)

Acknowledgements

Firstly I can't thank Kim and Sinclair Macleod of Indie Authors World enough for not only Kim's 'right when are you getting the book out' pressure, but their help and support, inspiration, ideas, and cover design from my 'I don't know what I want it to look like but here are a couple of images I like'. Thank you guys, this would not be real without you.

Lee Kayne of Saltire Books who got me started with some deadlines to get the initial content completed and his honesty to help me move forward with the project.

My mum for doing the editing, and along with my dad bringing me up to believe you can do anything you really want if you put your mind to it, the effort in and give your best effort all the way.

The Costello's Brian and Sheena for asking the painful questions, getting me through my bullshit excuses and basically being awesome friends that inspire and motivate me because they believe in me.

My friends, Grant, Susan, Sarah, Kirsty and Nicole (that is no particular order of importance) for not giving me shit for going AWOL while I was writing and believing and supporting me all the way.

The many people who read and reviewed chapters for me and the full book who I don't want start naming in case I miss and offend someone.

And the Universe for shaking things up, moving things in to my path, and creating the journey that has brought me to this point with knowledge and wisdom that I can share and help others.

ABOUT THE AUTHOR

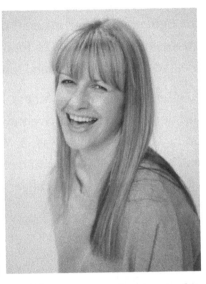

Jen Wilson (Sunday name Jennifer Margaret Wilson) has been working in the Health and Fitness industry since 2009. No one was more than surprised than herself over the industry she fell in love with, as a teen-ager she hated PE at school and would have done just about anything to try and get out of it. In her early 20's however she started to gain weight through her partying lifestyle and discovered the gym and fitness classes and started to see and like the changes she saw and had a desire to help others find something that fitted their life to help them improve their health and fitness.

A hobby became a passion and the passion became the desire for a new career. 2009 was the time to make that change and retrain. Since then she has gained qualifications in HND Fitness, Health and Exercise, BSc Sport and Exercise Science, PGDip TQFE and NLP Master Practitioner along with many industry relevant qualifications to teach the fitness classes and personal training that she loves. Away from teaching classes Jen strongly believes and lives a life where mindset is key focus before anything else. If your head is not in the right place then it makes it difficult and eventually impossible for the body to follow and that is why she created the Warrior Woman Project.

Outside of health and fitness Jen loves to travel and has been privileged to have travelled through parts of South East Asia, China, Russia, Mongolia, Australia and much of Europe and has grand plans to keep travelling. Life is very much about collecting experiences rather than stuff.

Her dream is to be able to reach as many women as possible with her no bullshit approach to health and happiness and teaching women that balance is key.

Connect with Jen at

E: jen@freedomintraining.co.uk

F: www.facebook.com/warriorwomanproject

T: www.twitter.com/warriorwomanJen

I: www.instagram.com/warriorwomanproject

W: www.warriorwomanproject.com

Lightning Source UK Ltd.
Milton Keynes UK
UKHW02f1004081117
312337UK00006B/250/P